CANCER:
IT'S NOT
A DEATH
SENTENCE

ROSS SUOZZI

CANCER: IT'S NOT A DEATH SENTENCE

THE STORY OF THREE FAMILY MEMBERS AND THEIR FIGHT TO DEFEAT CANCER

Printed in the United States of America.
ISBN: 978-1-94963-997-1
LCCN: 2019911316

Cover design by Carly Blake.
Layout design by George Stevens.

To the people we love.

To my mother, who lost her battle to ovarian cancer. The battle was long lost, as she waited too long to discover that her excessive belly fat was not what she thought. Possibly over a year went by without her seeking help. My mother holds a special place in my heart, and watching her be a princess on a pea pod in her last few months made for a memorable summary of her entire life.

To the caregivers who dedicate their lives to making the ones we love feel special and not forgotten during the battle. And to my sister, Anita, and brother-in-law, Tim, who dedicated their lives to making my mother comfortable. Watching how true devotion for love can make a delicate life ending a memory to cherish.

CONTENTS

INTRODUCTION 1

CHAPTER 1 5
Fighting Cancer

CHAPTER 2 23
Becoming a Cancer Caregiver

CHAPTER 3 43
Committing to Treatment

CHAPTER 4 55
Customizing Your Plan Based on What Matters Most

CHAPTER 5 75
Leading Your Team by Communicating Clearly

CHAPTER 6 93
Establishing a Trusting Relationship with Your Doctors

CHAPTER 7 107
Managing Your Pain

CHAPTER 8 125
Protecting Your Legacy

CHAPTER 9 139
Life after Cancer

INTRODUCTION

I f you're like me, you've spent your life reaching toward a vision of happiness that is meaningful to you, knowing full well that there are no guarantees that vision will become a reality. I do my best and put all my energy into work and family, but there is largely nothing I can do to prepare for an instantaneous change in which the ground just falls out from under my feet. None of us can be ready for that. And we shouldn't have to be. If we spent our days preparing for the worst, we wouldn't have any time or energy left to reach for our dreams. We'd probably also be crippled by anxiety and fear about the future.

Nevertheless, life-changing and life-threatening realities can come at us anytime, out of nowhere. Those realities recognize no distinctions among us. It doesn't matter who we are, what we do or have done, whom we know, or how we've lived our lives; any one of us can find ourselves suddenly facing a life-changing reality. Mine was cancer—my own, and then my wife's, and then our eldest son, Lorenzo's.

We turned to medical professionals, of course. But these were mostly strangers with no personal stake in our outcomes. I suspect there's an intentional disconnect built into the healthcare system for the purpose of keeping medical professionals objective and focused on their duties. Our medical staff was there to do a job to the best of their abilities, and that job was to come up with and implement treatment plans. However good their bedside manners may have been, their jobs were to stay focused on killing the thing that was threatening to kill each of us.

The doctors and nurses weren't there to give us special attention, coach us, or teach us everything we needed to know to survive each day, and they were most definitely not there to help us think about becoming and staying happy. They were working to keep our bodies alive, but it was up to each of us to keep our lives going. After diagnosis and during treatments, different aspects of each of our lives fell apart in ways that we had not anticipated. And we needed to learn quickly about things that we had never before thought we'd need to know.

For me, there was a horrible feeling that showed up alongside all the challenges posed by our cancers—that feeling became the impetus for this book. I decided to turn those trying experiences, moments of confusion and helplessness, and periods of utter loneliness into a guide for those of you facing cancer, whether your own or that of a close family member or friend. What you have in your hands now is the accumulated insight from the trial and error of my own cancer treatment, my wife's cancer treatment, and our eldest son's cancer treatment. We learned a lot, individually and as a family, from our experiences. Often, we learned what to do by suffering the consequences of not knowing beforehand. I want you to benefit from our experience, and I want both your treatment and your life to be as smooth as possible. I also want your treatment and your life to be truly yours, in the sense that I'd like you to know, right up front, that even though you are coping with cancer, you can absolutely still choose and be creative about how to live your life day to day.

Every type of cancer is different, and every person is different, which means that no two people are going to have identical experiences. That said, some things are true for us all, and one of them is that cancer treatment can leave you feeling empty and alone. The purpose of this book is to help you navigate and cope with that feeling, believe in yourself, and keep your friendships, your family, and your life intact while you work on kicking cancer's ass.

With cancer, as with life, there are a lot of factors we can't control. In my own battle with cancer, I learned that my job was to focus on the factors I *could* control, so that even if I was up against long odds, I could still bet on myself to win. Whatever someone has told you your odds are, I'll help you prepare yourself and help those around you make peace with what's happening and with what *may* happen. And if you're someone who is looking for ways to support a loved one with cancer, this book can help you too. I've been a patient and a caregiver—and learned a lot in each role. Your loved one will need your support, and these pages can give you some tools to coach them and you through this experience.

Cancer, and cancer treatment, saps time and energy. In this book, I make a case for using time wisely, for noticing daily opportunities to strengthen bonds with the people we're closest to, and for cutting out routines that we might have done out of habit but that didn't make us satisfied or happy. Figuring out what really matters and belongs in our lives is a critical step in battling cancer.

The first time you heard a doctor say, "It's cancer," it's likely that you felt helpless. For me, it was like I was suddenly heading toward the rapids in a leaky little boat without a paddle. I want you to know that you're not alone. I know these waters. I know it's going to be a lot of work, and it's going to get pretty rough at times, but together, we can do this.

CHAPTER 1

FIGHTING CANCER

I t was the afternoon before our brand-new gym facility was set to open its doors. My wife, Corinna, and I had designed the gym to meet the needs of our expanding clientele. I was up on a ladder, hanging television sets above the cardio center. Even though the pressure was still on us to get the last few items checked off the list, we could see our way to tomorrow, and we were thrilled to have made it this far. A little sheet metal here, some patina there, a couple more finishing touches near the entrance, and we'd be done for the night. I planned to bring in the equipment in the morning, and then we'd open the doors and welcome our members into their shiny new fitness center. I looked around me and saw eighteen thousand square feet of heaven.

I'd been coughing most of the day and had assumed that coughing was triggered by all the materials we'd been working with for so many weeks. With the last television set in hand, I carefully worked my way up the ladder with a cough rumbling in my chest and throat. I was coughing pretty hard the entire time I spent securing the set in the cradle and actually started struggling with my breath as I descended the ladder. When I reached the ground, I was having a full-on coughing fit—a bad one. By the time it finished, I was bent over, gripping the ladder with one hand and staring at the blood I'd just spat into the other. My thought at the moment was a strange one: "Come on, not now!" There was another coughing fit not long after that. And more blood.

I decided to call Corinna and explain that I wasn't coming home but was instead taking a trip to the emergency room—not an easy choice for me, given that I liked to think of myself as invincible. I had sucked up a lot of pain during the process of building our new gym, but this felt like a wake-up call to stop and get an expert opinion. By evening time, doctors were taking a bone marrow sample from my hip and running tests to see what was happening to me. I spent the better part of that evening in an urgent-care room and the entire next day in a hospital bed. Still, I wanted nothing more than to get on my feet and get our new gym opened. This was supposed to be one of the most important days of my life, and I was lying on my back, useless.

My wife, Corinna, made arrangements with a client of ours who had a moving company, and they got all the equipment into the building. By herself, Corinna completed the last bits of work and opened the new facility on time. Corinna would soon be running things by herself too, as I was repeatedly hospitalized for tests and transfusions.

* * *

Corinna and I had taken a huge leap of faith back when we decided to build a business. Though we both did other things professionally, we'd both also competed in body building competitions, so it was an enormous but natural step when we broke away from our corporate jobs to open a gym of our own. It was a lot of hard work, but we'd never been afraid of that, and it felt amazing to be our own bosses, doing what made us happy to get out of bed in the morning. In the 1950s, the American dream was a house with a white picket fence, but for us it was making a successful living doing what we enjoyed.

When we got our original business started, we'd rented a space and poured ourselves into every class, every training session, and every little detail. Our clients felt that devotion, and our little gym grew. After a handful of years, we grew out of the space we were leasing. Classes were getting a little too crowded, and the parking lot was always full. That was when we knew it was time for another leap of faith.

My previous profession had been working as a structural engineer and general contractor, and my knowledge from those jobs enabled us to design our own facility—one that would meet our present and future needs and that would be ours in a way that the rented property never was. We had an amazing core of members who supported our dream of creating the perfect building with state-of-the-art equipment, energizing classes, and an outdoor pool. We were going to build the new Peaks Athletic Club. We had the dream, the plans, and the encouragement from our clients, but we still needed the financing.

For that, we ended up having to go to *thirty-eight* banks. Yes, we had a thriving business. Yes, we had sound plans and plenty of know-how. But the financial climate was rough, and so many banks didn't want to take a risk on our small business. You'd have thought we were a couple of schoolkids trying to get a three-story building loan just to open a lemonade stand. I spent a thousand dollars printing copies of our proposal and assembling it in sleek binders to hand to each lender. Through all the rejections, we kept on making copies, assembling binders, and booking new appointments. We weren't about to let other people's (not even thirty-seven other people's) lack of faith in us shake our own.

When we did find a lender willing to work with us, instead of feeling great, it felt like entering into a deal with the devil. On the day we were signing the paperwork, with its every little detail laid out, Corinna's eyes caught mine and lingered there. I knew we were both thinking the same thing: once we signed all those documents, we wouldn't own anything anymore. The house we lived in with our two boys, our cars, the clothes we wore that day to assure the lender of our good intentions—the bank owned it all. Once we signed, the bank *owned us*.

We bought a little over one and a half acres of land in a great location, and construction got underway. Before too long, however, I brought it to a halt. Given my training, I had a better-than-average sense of when things just weren't right with a building. Things were most definitely not right. We had to fire the contractor who had botched the job. Then, that contractor tried to sue us for wrongful termination. Thankfully, the inspection findings proved me right. "The Great North Wall," as the family had nicknamed it, was eighteen inches too high and potentially in danger of falling over. Worse, it would have fallen across the property line, so the city had also started breathing down our necks to fix it.

We found a solution—a costly but effective way to anchor the base of the wall—but by then, we had another problem on our hands. Our bank didn't want to finish funding the project. Our rainy-day fund ended up being used to pay attorney's fees so we could *force* our lender to honor its commitment and let us get back to building. The construction site sat dormant for eight months while we fought with our own bank.

During the months battling the bank so that we could move forward toward the dream of owning our own space, I found what I thought was a spider bite on my left calf. It started as a raised area, and then it got an angry-looking ring around it. If you looked closely, you could see the flesh dissolving, which explains why I and the doctors thought my bite had come from a brown recluse spider. The bite got infected, so I got antibiotics for it; but not long after, I got another bite and then a third. The bites kept showing up in the same areas on my left calf, and the alleged bites would become infected extremely quickly.

More infections meant more antibiotics, and then more and more intense antibiotic prescriptions. We had started out with pills, and then moved to injections, and then to something called a "cannonball," which was essentially a grapefruit-sized container that we kept in the refrigerator. I could just open up the fridge and self-inject doses of antibiotic as necessary. My immune system eventually reacted negatively to the antibiotic as well as to the pain medicine that I'd been prescribed for my discomfort. So if I wanted to continue on the medicine, I needed to get used to breaking out in hives, having raw skin, and taking more medicines: anti-inflammatories and anti-histamines like Benadryl.

At one point, the nurse practitioner treating me suggested that I consult a hematologist to investigate a low white blood cell count, but I didn't listen. My eyes were on other things. They were just spider bites, and they were already a nuisance, given everything else that the family and I were dealing with. So instead of making an appointment with a hematologist, we called in a pest-control company to spray the house for spiders, and then we called it good.

* * *

After spending the night in the hospital and missing the opening of our new facility, I was able to get a blood transfusion to raise my white blood cell count—and I felt like a million bucks again. I was like a Tesla Roadster with a fresh charge. I nearly leapt out of bed, and I got right back to business like nothing had happened. As far as I was concerned, what happened was that I needed some new blood cells, and now I was all set.

That first night in the hospital coughing blood, my doctors acknowledged that I had more than a lingering infection. It became clear to them that I had a blood illness of some kind, but that really only opened the doors to them speculating about what precisely was going on. With no conclusive diagnosis of why my immune system was failing, the only solution was to restore the blood with transfusions. And with every transfusion, the new blood would ramp up my deficient immune system and give me the feeling that I was good to go, even "cured" for some time.

That feeling of being "cured" lasted for shorter and shorter amounts of time; like a car with increasingly bad gas mileage, my body was just eating up the blood. Naturally, my response to feeling weakened was to go back for another blood transfusion and another, until I'd started to need blood nearly every three days. The financial commitment got more intense the more frequently I needed a transfusion. At the time, just a single pint alone, without any of the other equipment or service, cost between $1,500 and $2,000. Our insurance didn't see those transfusions as necessary procedures, so we paid out of pocket for them. I'd be at the hospital, and I'd call Corinna over at the gym: "Baby, please sell some memberships today because I need some blood." Thankfully, because we were a new gym, she could actually sell those memberships, and then she would run over to the hospital and pay with cash for my transfusion.

Ultimately, I took *nineteen* pints of blood. That meant more money stress, more poor health, and eventually, more time in the hospital too. And hospital time meant more time on truly ugly pain-killers—synthetic morphine, fentanyl, and so many other opioids. I'll say more about pain medicine in later chapters, but for now, suffice it to say that although I couldn't function without the painkillers, I could barely function *with* them.

Corinna kept on top of everything during my hospital visits. She ran the business, took care of our two boys, and dealt with our hemorrhaging finances. Eventually, the doctors recognized that my immune system deficiency was so intense that they needed to run more tests. I didn't test positive for cancer at that point. What I con-clusively tested positive for, instead, was HIV.

Corinna went with me to the office of my hematologist and oncologist for that news about my lab results. Dr. Roberts came into the exam room and announced that there was information we needed to be aware of. With no hesitation whatsoever, he explained that I was HIV positive and that he would need to explore treatment for that result. I looked at Corinna and said, "Whatever you're thinking, don't. This can't be true!" My doctor suggested that we begin treatment right away. But I refused for a few reasons: first, the treatment is very invasive; second, at the time treatment for HIV cost around $12,000 a week; and third, I was convinced that I had cancer and not HIV. Instead of starting the HIV treatment, I proposed that the doctor give me some time to do research on my own.

Figuring there must be a reasonable explanation for that diagnosis, Corinna and I went home, and I started investigating false positive testing. My research showed that four people in one thousand receive false positives, and I determined that I must be one of those. For thirty days, though, I had an HIV diagnosis, until I insisted on and was able to get a more conclusive Western blot test. That test was $2,000 out of pocket, and it came back negative.

The days of living with the HIV diagnosis were brutal. I had been hiding, or trying to hide, being sick from our two boys, Lorenzo and Dominic. Besides making home life strange for them, my secretiveness about my illness also didn't help them much socially. I was a fairly high-profile figure in our little community, so when I would disappear for a few days or a couple of weeks at a time, people got to talking about what might be going on with me. Things got much worse when the HIV misdiagnosis was leaked by a lab technician who lived in our neighborhood and who went so far as to warn his own kids to stay away from Lorenzo and Dominic! From there, the rumors swirled: I was a junkie; I was a drug trafficker, and on and on.

It didn't help that those rumors carried weight in our community, where people were very concerned with keeping out any "bad elements." You might say that they were accustomed to a certain kind of successful living, and they were careful to have neighbors who reflected their values and their idea of success. Any suggestion that things were otherwise was enough to bring out people's insensitivity. Our adult neighbors had no trouble sharing that insensitivity with their own kids, which then made those kids feel emboldened to threaten and put down both Lorenzo and Dominic. We had to pull Lorenzo and Dominic out of school to keep them from being hazed by kids who were hearing bad things about their dad. That was hard on them, being uprooted and moved to a new school in Scottsdale. When I look back on it now, I feel lucky and thankful that this difficulty, one that affected our entire future as a family, only helped us to bond more closely together. Not every family might have had that same result.

* * *

It took about six more months before we went from "maybe it's cancer" to a tentative diagnosis of "a unique form of lymphoma." My body continued to deteriorate, and the lymph nodes in my arms and groin had grown enlarged and painful. Since there are over one hundred varieties of lymphoma, I had to be treated generally, while the doctors—a whole team of them communicating with specialists at the Mayo Clinic, the MD Anderson Center, and another clinic in Albuquerque—worked to determine the precise type.

Still, I continued to struggle with the idea that this was supposed to have been the time of our lives. Corinna and I had worked our asses off to get where we were, and I wasn't about to accept that the universe was now knocking me onto mine. Corinna had emigrated from England; my grandparents had moved their lives from Italy eighty years prior, and this was the moment when we had expected to experience the result of all the work we and our families had done to build a better life. Instead of feeling like we were achieving our goals, our expectations had come to a screeching halt because my body had decided to quit. That physical deterioration was an experience I was far from familiar with. I had put a lot of effort into my health and my physique, and I think that made it even more difficult for me to process what was happening. This was my first experience with being physically challenged. And damn, what a reality check; I went from feeling invincible to feeling helpless.

Lymphoma was a word I absolutely did not want to hear. It was also definitely not a word I wanted our bank to hear. The pressure from our bank hadn't let up once the new facility opened. If anything, that pressure intensified. The bank called us

Lymphoma was a word I absolutely did not want to hear.

every day to ask for numbers: "What were your sales today?" or "How many people worked out there today?" It didn't take us long to realize that, with the building finished and opened, our lenders felt they could make more money by selling it to another, bigger fitness organization. For that, they needed us to fail. They didn't want our interest payments on the loan. They wanted us to close so they could sell the building out from under us. That meant we would receive "friendly" check-in conference calls from them every single day.

Sometimes, I was in a hospital bed for three days, sometimes three weeks. I took a lot of those daily conference calls from inside the hospital. I would take the phone into the tiny bathroom inside my hospital room, because I didn't want the lenders to hear doctors being paged, hall-wide announcements, or the beeping equipment in my room. So there I was in the bathroom, hopped up on opioids, hunched over the phone in my hospital gown, attempting to reassure our lender that everything was great at the gym. Those guys at the bank were sharks, circling in the water, and I was badly wounded. I felt strongly that I needed to do whatever I could to keep from being attacked.

Our lenders did learn about my illness eventually. At one point, the bank agent in charge of making our lives more difficult actually told me that I was at a point in my life where I'd "reached the end of my personal capacity." He effectively told me to lie down and die, which only raised my determination to defy him.

* * *

I started chemotherapy during the time that we were working with the diagnosis of "a type of lymphoma." I remember that first chemo treatment, and in a way, it was a microcosm of my whole cancer treatment experience.

It was some time in the middle of the night when the hospital nurses woke me up to give me the treatment. I was half asleep and half out of my mind from the fentanyl, so I could hardly make sense of what was happening. About all I understood was what I saw and felt: the nurse hooked my arm to what looked like a gallon freezer bag full of murky, colorless fluid, and it burned as it went in. It was like the feeling of pouring rubbing alcohol on an open wound, except that the burning sensation went through my veins and all the way up my arm. I begged for more painkillers to help me cope. I was confused, in pain, and all alone except for when the nurse came back to hook up a second bag. That one was a pretty, red-colored fluid.

That first chemo experience was more or less what the rest of treatment was like for me: alone, half out of my mind from pain-killers, unsure of what was happening, and uninformed about what was coming next. The experience of chemotherapy was inconsistent. In most cases, patients will schedule treatment at a local infusion center with a weekly schedule for the entire round prescribed by the oncologist. My experience differed immensely; the state of my health dictated how and when the infusion would be administered. When I could have outpatient infusions, special precautions would be necessary.

Because of my immune system deficiency, I had to wear a mask to the chemo infusion center and stay put in a little isolated corner while there. Sometimes, a single chemo treatment had to be split over two consecutive days, because my veins just couldn't handle the volume of fluid. But the other cancer patients at the center—people who were going through some terrible and scary stuff—were lucid. They were socializing, watching television, even knitting. I'd be sitting there for eight hours at a time, and I'd watch those people come and go after two hours, maybe even after only forty-five minutes.

It's lousy, I know, to have compared my cancer and my suffering to others'. But there I was, practically drooling on myself, and through my fog, I envied them.

After I'd withstood generalized treatments for far too long, my doctors were able to cross-reference a few different blood test results and finally come up with a proper diagnosis: non-Hodgkin lymphoma. That gave the medical team what they needed for a more focused course of treatment, but to me, it was all still a mystery. I didn't know what that meant for my prognosis or how my treatments might change.

> *After I'd withstood generalized treatments for far too long, my doctors were able to cross-reference a few different blood test results and finally come up with a proper diagnosis: non-Hodgkin lymphoma.*

* * *

Corinna was busy filling every void in our business and household activities. I was scrambling to keep my life moving forward. And there were two young active boys demanding that I be there as a father for them when I was capable. Lorenzo and Dominic really didn't have an understanding of my complete condition, but they still had a plan to spend time together with me.

The boys had this wild dream of buying a boat. They were earning money by working as parking lot attendants, parking cars for the Fountain Hills Art Fair. At ten and twelve, they were making something like five dollars a car, and it all went into this big burlap sack. They didn't spend it on candy, comic books, or other obvious kid things. It all went into the bag. They kept working and saving, and that bag kept getting heavier.

During my hospital stays, the boys would have to wear these clean-room suits and masks to visit me, but they'd just sit around my hospital bed like everything was cool. I would have them pick up a *Boat Trader* magazine, and we'd circle ads for boats they wanted to look at. Eventually they saved up $1,500. I was really impressed by their commitment. They wanted a boat, and they'd taken personal responsibility for earning money and figuring out how to get one.

I'd figured that, realistically, they'd end up with a canoe or maybe a paddle boat. Nope. One day when we were home together, they circled a nineteen-foot long Sea Ray—a serious pleasure boat—and said, "Let's go get it!" I was feeling rough, but I drove the boys over to the seller's house that same day. The boat had been sitting for too long and had some cosmetic damage, but it was sound. The guy selling it wanted $4,000 for it. My sons did something I'd never seen them do either before or since: they batted their eyes and looked so sad. "But our dad has cancer!" And then they explained our family's experience to him.

Dominic and Lorenzo produced their big sack of money and pushed it into the seller's hands. The guy looked at my boys, at me standing half dead in his driveway, and then he looked at the money bag and asked how much was in it. They told him it was about $1,500. He took a deep breath and accepted the deal. We hitched up the boat and drove home, the boys all the while admiring their purchase through the rearview mirror. After that, cleaning and readying the Sea Ray became our father-and-sons activity. Once it was all reupholstered and polished up, our plan was to take it out fishing.

* * *

We had our goals for the boat, but it was going to be quite a while before we could achieve them. My veins had gotten severely deteriorated from multiple treatments. I'd had a series of PICCs and ports put into my skin for the infusions, and these had to be removed whenever they got infected. Over and over again, they kept getting infected. And then there was one day when the treatment pushed an infection right up into my heart. I collapsed and lost consciousness.

When I woke up, I was in the cardiac ward, one-on-one with a nurse, being told that I wasn't going to make it through the night. My wife was there, and the look in her eyes frightened me. After all we'd been through up to this moment, hearing the doctor say that I was pretty much already dead and had little chance of making it through the night was just too much for her. She left that night, and I had this awful fear in my gut that she wasn't going to be back. I had never seen that look in her eyes before.

The depth of her fear was overwhelming; even to this day, I remember that night as the *only* time Corinna showed true fear of my condition. At one point later in the evening, there was a priest, or maybe the hospital chaplain, hovering around my door. I knew that he was there to help me make my peace with dying. I told him he was not welcome. I'd love to say that I was nicer about it than that, but I was in no shape or mood to be polite. Everyone was ready for me to die but me. I'm sure everyone assumed that I was in denial, as I had been at so many moments leading up to this point. But they were wrong. That night I felt something different—something less like denial and more like determination. I remember thinking I'd come too far in my life and worked too hard for the things I wanted and believed in. I was going to be with my wife. I was going to raise my boys. I was going to enjoy my hard-won successes.

That night, I had nothing but a hospital crash cart for company.

It felt like everybody gave up on me. That's when I decided that I was going to work on living. I remember thinking, "I have too much shit going on, and I am not ready to die yet!" This was the defining moment when I realized that cancer was not my death sentence. I requested that the nurse check every fifteen minutes to make sure that I was awake. Even though I was loaded up with fentanyl, my heart rate bumping at 175 beats per minute, I was determined not to have a junkie's dream experience. My plan was to stay awake for the entire night, and my only goal in that moment

This was the defining moment when I realized that cancer was not my death sentence.

was to be in control of my life. I spent the rest of that long, lonely night doing nothing but breathing. It took every bit of effort I could muster. Breathe in. Breathe out. My entire night, my entire life had that singular focus. Breathe in. Breathe out. That's how I made it through to sunrise. This particular night and this task changed my entire life. It defined who I can be for the rest of my life. The challenge I endured raised the bar on what I could achieve if all other distractions could be eliminated and a focus of attention is directed into one important, meaningful endeavor.

* * *

In later chapters, I'll share more details of my experiences with diagnosis and treatment, but what I most want to say to you now is something I don't think gets said often enough, and it's this: there is very likely going to be some mystery when it comes to your own cancer diagnosis and treatment. There will be very many variables that will need to be taken into account, some elements will remain unknown, and others will not be definitively determined at any point.

We may live in a world where we've come to expect immediate information and service, but with cancer, answers still aren't immediately available. It takes time to resolve some of the questions and complications that inevitably arise, whether during diagnosis or during treatment itself. It might take two weeks before your test results are produced, and then those results may be communicated to you in a speedy, prerecorded telephone message.

When we're seeking answers and seeking help, it is very, very easy to have intense emotional reactions to every- and anything. We can easily become frustrated, angry, fearful. Even if we're someone who usually has their shit together, all the mysteries, the confusion, the testing, and all the time those take can easily make us go a little crazy. I think it's fair to say that you're going to get emotional throughout this process. And you're also probably going to feel isolated and even lonely. This may be the time in your life to examine the inner you. Learn more about your behavior and reactions. Even if you have a solid support system in place, not everybody can be with you every step of the way. What I am here to tell you is that there is a way through those feelings of helplessness in relation to the mystery of it all, of loneliness through all the hours of all the days that you have to survive, and even through the pitfalls of anger, frustration, and other overwhelming emotions. The way through those feelings depends on you figuring out some things, the first of which is figuring out how to believe in yourself enough to push through all the truly uncomfortable stuff that's coming your way.

Becoming a cancer warrior requires some specific traits that your inner awareness needs preparation for. The inner shadow now has easy exposure to your persona; with this said, all the pent-up negative emotions—including rage, envy, and fear—could surround your entire day. I point this out, as my experience was dominated by my shadow. The internal struggle I endured battled to suppress my shadow and bury it to save my own life. Your cancer warrior needs awareness and openness for the real fight to save your life. I plan to share the tools needed to succeed, the tools your medical team will not supply you with. This experience cannot be taught unless one has succeeded for oneself.

In chapter 3, we'll get into the details of consciously choosing to believe in yourself, but right now, I want to tell you a little bit about Corinna and Lorenzo.

CHAPTER 2

BECOMING A CANCER CAREGIVER

My year of treatment for lymphoma was the hardest and scariest time of my life. And after that year, there were still a lot of adjustments to be made. My body still looked like my body, though I'd lost a lot of weight. I would tell people that it felt like getting into your car to discover that somebody swapped out the V-8 for a four cylinder. Sure, it still looks like the same car, but it doesn't quite act or feel like it. After working so hard for so many years to develop my physique—chasing a vision of physical perfection—it was really hard for me to accept my new limitations. There's no point in pretending that I never felt down about not being in fighting trim anymore.

My eyesight had changed from chemo. The intravenous antibiotics I took for the "spider bites" had given me every side effect in the literature. From my knees down, tendons and ligaments weren't what they used to be, and I couldn't perform the way I wanted. My durability was drastically reduced too. I could do something strenuous and feel like my old self again for a little while, but then I'd be in bed or on the couch for the next three days recovering.

It's no wonder that my family was looking at me differently—like I was made of glass—and had changed the way they interacted with me. After such a prolonged period of illness, it was like they didn't trust that I was really better. They were worried that I'd relapse or get sick again with something else, and I felt like they'd gotten used to thinking of me as a sick person. I didn't want to be viewed as an invalid or constantly see pity in my loved ones' eyes. With people always asking what they could do for me, it was difficult to keep from feeling tense and answering, "Leave me alone."

I spent much of that time following treatment learning to adjust, to adapt to what I could do *now*, instead of letting myself fall into self-pity and bemoan the loss of my ability to do what I *used to* be able to do. The past may have been good, but I needed to learn to live in the present. My wife was amazing, and I really clung to her for support. It meant everything to me to always have her to count on. I came to see what I had otherwise taken for granted—all the very specific things that Corinna would do to make our lives run as smoothly as possible. The business and household chores, the small but significant acts of parenting, the finished laundry so soft and clean smelling. We had already developed a sturdy support structure together as parents and business owners, but now we had really learned to dance together in this well-choreographed routine. After two years or so, I started feeling like life was pretty much back to normal. Well, it was the new normal anyway. The adjustments were getting easier to handle, and the whole family was starting to relax.

* * *

Corinna went in for a routine gynecologist visit—and that's when they found several "concerning" lumps. We spent days worrying and wondering what was coming next. The doctors did their biopsies and lab work and then diagnosed Corinna with midstage cervical cancer.

It hardly seemed possible. Initially, all I could think was, "Not again." I was angry. After all we'd been through with my lymphoma, it was horrible to accept that now my wife was in for a battle with *another* form of cancer. I struggled to imagine how we would go through that process again. One thing we knew, though, was that this time, we needed a better plan of action. We had to get good answers to all our questions and get a correct diagnosis quickly. I became determined to use my personal experience with treatment to make this ordeal easier and better for Corinna.

> I learned from personal experience that lost time is lost opportunity, so we moved straight to treatment.

We also didn't linger in denial this time, as I'd done when I was trying to put Band-Aids on my own health problems and pretend they'd eventually go away. I learned from personal experience that lost time is lost opportunity, so we moved straight to treatment. And since we already had the problem pinpointed, Corinna started with the correct course of treatment.

As worried as we were that she was going to suffer the same way I had, her experiences were unique. We learned that just as every form of cancer is different, the treatments would be too. Corinna had chemo, but she had radiation also, and her treatments were nearly all outpatient procedures. That meant that Corinna spent most nights at home in her normal environment. Her longest hospital stay was for two nights when she had abdominal pains and was kept for observation. Having her at home through those seven months made a big difference to the well-being of our family both emotionally and, as any of you who have ever had to pay for hospitalization already know, financially. There were times when Corinna had pain, but hers wasn't constant as mine had been, and we were both grateful for that. She avoided opioid painkillers and all the difficulties they present, including the threat of addiction.

Nevertheless, worry was a huge part of my life during Corinna's treatment. Being the one who's sick, I learned, is a very different experience from being the spouse or loved one of a person with cancer. I was scared for her constantly. This was the woman I loved most in the world; witnessing her fighting for her life had me distressed for months.

* * *

I'd relied on Corinna's support and help during and after my own treatment, and I was determined to be there for her in every way possible. This time it was *my* job to make sure *she* stayed positive, to keep things going with our business, and to make sure the boys were well taken care of. Being on the other side of that coin was eye-opening, particularly to the ways in which caregiving is very tough work. I learned that I needed to be emotionally tuned in to her as much as I was task oriented. I could complete the chores fairly well (though my laundry never turned out as fluffy as Corinna's), but the emotional side was far more challenging. Sometimes the focus was a daily ailment; other times it was the digestion of new medical news. Still other times we would work together on just finding a comfortable "normal" state.

Just like when I was the patient—but now as the patient's support person—I needed to develop some mental and emotional toughness to get through Corinna's treatment and recovery. I worked on being mindful, but I struggled to keep my shit together, which I realized is pretty impossible to do when your loved one is suffering. I guess I saw it as part of my job as a caregiver to hide (or at least try to hide) my expression of intense emotions without also seeming to be evasive or seem like I was trying to hide the truth.

There were many occasions when I understood new medical news before Corinna did, and frequently I would shed a tear before she or our sons could see. I felt that I needed to hide at least some of my emotions to prevent the rest of the family from overreacting to bad news and to keep myself together so that I could care for them. For me, that meant forming a thick skin or a kind of mask.

For example, during Corinna's treatment, there was a procedure called brachytherapy that she had to undergo as part of her radiation regimen. As the doctor explained the procedure to us, he demonstrated how a probe would be inserted into the vagina, and a quick burst of radiation would be shot precisely in the direction of the cancer tissue. Corinna insisted that I be there for the procedure, and to our surprise, the procedure wasn't exactly as the doctor had described it. The doctor had left out some key details. Corinna was medicated but awake, and a cloth barrier had been set up so that she could not see what was actually going on between her legs. The machine was large, a Frankenstein-looking contraption, and the probe itself enough to make a porn star second-guess its purpose. Corinna was pretty uncomfortable after they inserted the probe, and she kept asking me for reassurance. I looked her in the eye and explained that everything was fine, though we were both more than ready for the radiation to get underway and be finished.

Then the doctor explained that he was now ready to pack Corinna's womb with gauze pads, and he opened a sterile bag that looked to me like it contained enough pads to absorb an MMA fighter's blood. That's when Corinna's pain went to level 10, and she squeezed my hand harder than I knew she had the strength to do. I could not believe how much gauze had to be forced into her, even though it was a necessary part of protecting the surrounding tissue from being irradiated. I knew that I needed to be her strongest support in that moment, and yet there I was, completely shocked by what was happening to her. That might have been the most helpless I've ever felt in my life. I think that one of the really hard parts of being a caregiver is being torn between your own shock and distress and the need to be strong for the ones you love. Needless to say, I did my best to mask, or at least quiet, my own emotional response so that I could help Corinna through the pain and distress of that event.

I think that one of the really hard parts of being a caregiver is being torn between your own shock and distress and the need to be strong for the ones you love.

For all the work we did to be sure that Corinna's experience of treatment wouldn't involve some of the pitfalls of my own, we faced complications and challenges that were unique to her form of cancer. For one thing, instead of having a single oncologist to form a working relationship with, we had a team of specialists, each prescribing and performing different treatments. That meant we were in a different outpatient facility five days a week. She had chemo on Mondays and various forms of radiation each day for the rest of the week. Every day was a different treatment method at a different location; it almost felt like we were just spinning a big wheel to see what and where her treatment would be on any given day.

Because there were multiple physicians, we had multiple personalities to navigate, and not all of them were especially good at explaining the treatments. One lesson we hadn't quite learned from my experience was to ask as many questions as we needed to. We mostly just accepted the advice we were given and took the prescribed steps; I think that was partly why we felt like we didn't quite know what was coming next. Treatment was still pretty mysterious, and the vague descriptions we were given for treatment methods weren't much help when it came to making sure we were emotionally prepared.

So if we'd asked more questions when we learned that Corinna would be having "internal radiation," we might have arrived for her treatment better prepared for exactly what Corinna would experience. Instead, we went in relatively blind. Corinna might not have had to lie there with tears in her eyes for hours while she got her prescribed dose of direct radiation. She might not have had to feel so uncomfortable or humiliated, and I might have been a better support to her during the procedure.

For all our attempts to be prepared, we simply didn't know all the questions we needed to ask. On the one hand, we needed to trust her physicians. On the other hand, we needed to be the ones who were looking after our own mental and emotional well-being. Ultimately, that meant getting savvy, and sometimes courageous, about talking to doctors. It was a challenge to figure out what information we needed and didn't yet have, but we learned that if we heard something that didn't make sense to us, or if we felt like we didn't understand, we really needed to stop and ask questions until things started to become clear.

* * *

Corinna's treatments would leave her feeling worn down and weak, depleted of every ounce of energy. She spent nearly every day feeling only half alive. When she underwent radiation, she said she could smell both the radiation treatment and the dead skin cells afterward. Chemo left her nauseous and vomiting, and her bodily waste would smell odd afterward. Her schedule was to get chemo each Monday and radiation the days after that. After Monday, she would feel trashed for the next three days as her body processed all that poison. Even after those days passed, she'd be exhausted from the aftereffects of the chemo and from all the other treatments that week. Then the whole process would start all over again the next Monday. Because she felt badly every day, it became difficult for Corinna to stay positive. That meant we had to think seriously about lifestyle changes that would benefit her.

Corinna wanted to formulate a plan early, and her specific goal was to keep her body from wasting. If you're not familiar with wasting, it is a debilitating process in which the body causes its own muscle tissue and fat to waste away. Corinna witnessed how deteriorated my body had become during and after treatment, and so her primary goal was to ensure that she maintained an active lifestyle during her entire treatment.

We both already knew how common it is for cancer patients to feel like they've just had enough. When each day is its own unique struggle, it's surprisingly easy to think that there's not any point in continuing on. When my physical and mental capacity reached their low points, it was as if it were happening for the first time in my life; I didn't know that I was capable of experiencing feeling that low. The uncertainty and mystery of cancer makes it difficult to distinguish among the choices available. And then there is the suffering and the pain that follows and further complicates things. The first and easiest option is to surrender and quit, but Corinna and I both knew that with careful consideration, we could muster the tenacity to choose the more difficult option, which is to persevere and not give up. Mustering that effort felt a lot like a last-ditch effort, a final attempt to defend ourselves against both the disease and the treatment.

You'll remember me saying earlier that this is just the sort of thing for which the medical community does not assist its patients. When it comes to the medical aspects of your treatment, there is no time or space for the mental and emotional needs that arise, and actually treating those needs may not be something that is covered by your insurance. That does not mean there are no options, but you may have to actively seek them out—things like cancer support groups, individual counseling, and partnering with a peer who has experienced the same type of cancer you have. What Corinna and I learned together, and what we know can be true for you, too, is that we all have in us more determination and perseverance than we might have expected. Corinna and I also learned and practiced some strategies for keeping our eyes on our goals of surviving cancer. That means we both know that there is a way for you to keep your eye on the prize too. You may be in a cloudy mental state, and the variables may be so numerous that you cannot imagine getting a handle on them even in your best health. But if you can focus, formulate a plan, and remind yourself of the lifestyle you once enjoyed, you can hold on to that goal as a means of pushing through your darkest hours. For Corinna, one simple but very serious goal was to ride her mountain bike again. She so enjoyed taking that bike out for a weekly ride that getting back on and riding once again was an aim she could hold on to.

When Corinna hit her low point, I could see what she was going through, could see how hard it was for her, and there was nothing I could do that could just fix things. That's what I most wanted—to fix things for her. As a caregiver, I struggled to follow my own idea that it was important to focus on the time beyond her treatment and recovery. I wanted most to keep in mind that once Corinna was past this, she could get back to the things she loved, even if on different terms. As her caregiver, I felt I needed to keep focused on her recovery so that I could help her focus on the time beyond treatment.

* * *

This is where the learning curve is steep when it comes to caring for a loved one, and the challenges can potentially take you down. That's why I think that being a caregiver absolutely requires a deeply optimistic approach to life. I also think that this deep optimism may be an emotional skill or attitude that new caregivers have no experience with. As caregivers, I think we feel right away the demand to be deeply optimistic, but the fact is that we have little time to practice our optimism before we are required to act. There is no pause button on life, no avoidance of what each day brings, no time to brush up on our skills. And yet, with each day, a caregiver's focus cannot drift in a direction other than the goal of a successful recovery; I really believe that it is up to the caregiver to stick to the patient's plans for recovery—even more than the patient.

For me, I had to learn that my urge to fix things was not even part of what real optimism demanded. Corinna helped me see that sometimes the best I could do for her, emotionally, was to acknowledge the awfulness of her treatment so that she would feel listened to and understood. I absolutely still did what I could to get her to entertain the idea of full recovery and cancer-free living, but part of what it meant to do that was to be there with her to accept her experience and her pain. From my point of view, having survived my own year of treatment, I wanted her to know that when she got back to living her life more fully, these hardships would eventually fade. I wholeheartedly believed—and continue to believe—that what we needed was to bravely endure the most difficult moments, to get through another day of pain and discomfort and get closer to her goal.

There may be a point in your caregiving task where it becomes extremely clear that recovery is not attainable. But that does not change the need for you to be supportive. I encourage you and, should you have them, your team of family and friends to find a way to take a positive approach to the precious time your loved one may have. My family's experience has shown us that difficult times are made easier if they are filled with what is most meaningful to us. Maybe your role as a caregiver will be to help formulate a wish list or a "bucket list" of things your loved one would like to do once again or for the first time. Walking in the park, eating a favorite meal— these can be the comforts that people need to have some balance and sense of comfort in their lives. Whatever these are, they should be front and center in your mind.

* * *

The boys and I tried to put some fun back into Corinna's days and keep her spirits up. She needed an escape from the grind of her treatment, so we tried to provide some little diversions doing things she enjoyed. Those diversions were anything that would get us away from home for a bit, including a ride to the mountains, spending some time on the lake altogether, maybe a weekend trip to a cabin. When Corinna said she wanted to go to a convention in Las Vegas, it sounded to me like a great idea. I wanted her to have a weekend away to just feel normal and enjoy life a little, and I wanted to keep her spirits up and keep her mind-set positive. We bought tickets to the Fitness Trade Show and made the room reservation, and our minivacation from the drudgery of cancer treatment was underway. From Phoenix to Las Vegas is about a five-hour drive, so I took the wheel, and away we went.

Five hours in a car was five hours too many. I might have remembered the time that I contracted pneumonia by going into the mountains during my own treatment, but I didn't. It hadn't sunk in for either of us yet that sometimes even "a little escape" can just be too much to handle in a treatment-weakened state. Just the movement of the car for five hours was too much for Corinna. It caused serious inflammation and irritation of her internal organs. All we wanted was to get her out of the house and do something special. But because we tried to do too much too soon, we set her health back.

What I hadn't quite learned as a patient, and what I still had to learn as a caregiver, was that the little things that seem so ordinary when we're well can be too much to deal with when we're undergoing treatment. A simple trip to the grocery store may seem harmless enough, but it may be rough going with an immune system that is weakened or compromised. Think about how many people are wandering around out there in the world, picking things up, putting them down again, coughing, sneezing, and so forth. Sometimes an outing into "normal life" isn't what's needed to get better. With Corinna, staying in a more stable, controllable environment would have been best. By trying to do too much, we delayed her return to that normal life we all wanted for her.

* * *

After a rough seven months, Corinna completed treatment and successfully joined the family of cancer survivors. She had to make the same sorts of adjustments that I did after treatment. She couldn't perform athletically at the same level that she had before and had to make peace with her altered body. And so, for a time, we adjusted to our lives as they were, and we did it together. Stairs brought on aches and pains that they hadn't before. Our workouts weren't the same as they were, but we kept at it. We honestly couldn't imagine giving them up. Exercise made us glad to roll out of bed every day. We knew that it would be nearly impossible to return to the physical condition we were in before our cancers took hold. We worked on being thankful that we still had our bodies, our family, and our business. We worked on believing that life was good and that we were far from done with it.

At the same time that we entertained those positive thoughts, we also walked on eggshells again and for a long time after Corinna's treatment. The boys were still pretty young, so we were, all four of us, still living together as a family at the time. And just as it had after my year of treatment, every sniffle got a worried look. If any one of us sneezed or coughed, the rest of our eyes were on that person immediately. Corinna and I had lost the confidence that had come along with our formerly robust health. We were afraid that one of us would take another sudden turn for the worse. Still, we adjusted, and life settled back into its normal patterns. The pull of those patterns was so strong, as was our hopefulness for a normal life, that five years after I had lymphoma and three years after Corinna's cervical cancer, we were once again shocked by what happened with Lorenzo, our oldest son.

* * *

Lorenzo was nineteen at the time; he was going to college and had lived in his own place for about six months. During his late teenage years, Lorenzo had some mild breathing issues and swollen tonsils.

We made the usual visits to the family doctor, but at no point did anyone think that Lorenzo's issues were anything serious. Neither we nor Lorenzo's doctors even entertained the idea of a blood test to see if that could help explain why he wasn't feeling 100 percent.

One weekend, Lorenzo and a friend visited friends of theirs who lived near our house, and so the two of them stayed at our place that Saturday night. Lorenzo woke up feeling weak and ill. He'd been fine the night before but had clear flu-like symptoms in the morning. His deterioration that morning was quick, and soon enough, we were in the emergency room in the same hospital where my wife and I had received our diagnoses.

We walked into the emergency room, and a doctor recognized me and my last name. He asked, "Is that your son in there?" I told him it was, and the look on his face brought back all my distress from when Corinna was sick. Lorenzo's bloodwork was abnormal, and the doctor had suspected that Lorenzo might have mono. But having seen that Lorenzo was my son, and considering my history, the doctor became convinced that the diagnosis for Lorenzo was leukemia.

I felt like my entire life changed again in that moment. Hearing that I had cancer was awful, and hearing that my wife had cancer was even worse. But my feelings about Lorenzo's condition were entirely new. Just the day before, Lorenzo had been a bright, healthy college student with his whole life ahead of him. Not even twenty-four hours later, I was consumed with worry that we were going to lose him. The aggressiveness of his form of leukemia was like nothing either Corinna or I had ever seen or experienced. His symptoms came on so suddenly and with such vengeance. That morning, my expectations were that Lorenzo would receive a treatment for the flu or possibly bronchitis. Even mono would have been fantastic. But leukemia?

Lorenzo wasn't even coherent. He was babbling, unresponsive, and otherwise just lying there hunched over in pain. The sudden change is his disposition was quick, and it looked like he was dying right in front of us. We didn't know if we needed to start preparing for the worst, but we also felt like we weren't going to let the worst happen without putting up a fight. My first thought was to contact the oncologist who had assisted me through my lymphoma, but it turned out that Lorenzo's case was beyond that doctor's specialty training. So he referred us to a young doctor who had just joined his Arizona oncology group, and that doctor, Dr. Abbas, came to the hospital on Sunday night to meet us.

Dr. Abbas examined Lorenzo, who was still unresponsive and bent over in pain on his hospital bed. After finishing the examination, Dr. Abbas asked us, "So what's his problem?" I thought that was a pretty wild question! *Leukemia* was his problem, right? "Sure," Dr. Abbas said, "but why is he curled up in a fetal position?" That wasn't normal? This was the first we were hearing about it. Just as we were thinking that our boy might be even worse off than we thought, the doctor said, "Don't worry. I'll have your son up out of that bed in two hours. He'll be walking around and talking to you. Two hours." Hearing him say that was an incredible relief. It was like somebody had just opened a window, and we only then realized that we'd been suffocating.

Pretty soon Lorenzo had a cocktail of medications in him, and sure enough, he was up and walking around again. He was talking to us, and for the first time since he'd been admitted earlier that day, he looked like he wasn't going to die on the spot. True to his word, Dr. Abbas had Lorenzo up and on his feet within two hours. It seemed like a miracle to us. It was the break we were hoping for and one we certainly wish for every parent—that the universe might grant relief to their sick child. This relatively sudden return to normal was the sort of simple thing that I know most people would trade their fortunes for. On many occasions, I have heard other families explaining that they would spend any amount of money they have to heal their child. And here was our son looking alive again from a simple steroid, some pain reliever, something for nausea, and so on. It was symptom relief, but it seemed miraculous.

Lorenzo was actually annoyed with us for the way we were all staring at him, wide-eyed and freaked out. He was feeling so much himself again that the attention was making him self-conscious and irritable. He didn't even want to let into the room some of the friends we'd called because he could see that they were visibly upset. So Lorenzo announced that he was taking a shower, and he shut the bathroom door behind him.

How different this was from trying to get my own diagnosis years earlier! Lorenzo was diagnosed the same night he came in, and within a week, we had a doctor who was obviously more than a match for the disease. I know that there were other factors, not the least of which was that Lorenzo had leukemia, but both Corinna and I were amazed at the advances that had been made in the years since that afternoon when I had started spitting up blood. Here we were, *ten* years past that day, and great advances had been made. There were better diagnostic tools, more treatments available, and more reasons to hope than ever.

With Lorenzo's treatment, our lives changed again. Corinna and I were old hands by then at supporting a loved one with cancer, but this time cancer came with different challenges and responsibilities that, once again, we hadn't really thought about until they were right on top of us. We had to make sure that Lorenzo was withdrawn from all his classes so that his college professors wouldn't just fail him for not showing up. At college, it's the student's responsibility to take care of these sorts of things or to deal with the consequences of an F or an Incomplete on their transcript and the loss of registration priority that comes with it. Lorenzo also had rent and utility bills at his place, and the time for us to figure out what was necessary was short. Credit cards, car payments—we needed to be proactive in order to keep things from falling apart while Lorenzo worked on getting better. Goals for his care were established very early, because we needed his recovery to be his number one job.

* * *

Lorenzo's treatment was very different from what either Corinna or I had undergone. He took chemotherapy treatments both in and out of the hospital like me, and radiation treatments like Corinna's, but there were bone marrow transplants too. There was a whole hospital floor dedicated to the department where they treated him. Sanitary conditions had improved greatly, and all visitors were required to wash their hand before they even entered the isolated floor. There were cleansing stations at the entrances and exits, so outside contaminants weren't as big a concern as they'd been for me.

Lorenzo's treatment included full-body radiation; instead of a focused spot treatment, he would walk into this special room, sort of like a vault. They would seal him in, and he'd be in there alone for an hour getting irradiated from all sides. It was like he was standing in a giant microwave. That experience could have been a lot worse for the entire family, except that this time around, his treatments were explained to us so much better than our own treatments had been.

The advancements that had been made in treatment options were obvious, but so were the ways treatments were explained and scheduled. It wasn't great knowing that he'd be in the hospital on his birthday, or on another holiday, but at least we knew it was going to happen, and we could plan for it. Corinna and I showed up to Lorenzo's appointments resolved to ask our every question, but nearly all the details were already laid out for us. The whole process was so much more structured than what we'd been through, and there was far less mystery about what was going to happen at each phase of Lorenzo's treatment. The entire culture of cancer treatment had undergone a serious overhaul.

We were pleasantly surprised by these improvements, of course, but that didn't stop us from being the caregivers who asked a thousand questions and sometimes challenged the doctors. One way that we challenged Lorenzo's medical team was when it came to pain relief options. Leukemia is painful, and we didn't want him suffering through the bombardment of opioids that I had. With Lorenzo being only nineteen, the risk of addiction was very real to us, and we felt like we needed to take significant action to keep that from happening. I asked Lorenzo's pain management doctor to provide him medical marijuana, and the doctor agreed. He put Lorenzo on a responsible dosage of synthetic, capsulized THC called Marinol, and that really did the job very well.

Some of Lorenzo's friends used marijuana on a recreational basis. Instead of frowning on it, like many parents might have done in other circumstances, we saw that it actually seemed to help keep Lorenzo's spirits up to have a party atmosphere in his room. Since the odds for surviving leukemia are a little better than a coin toss, we wanted to do every little thing we could to make his time in the hospital better. We also believed that he would be a lot more likely to live if he actually *wanted* to.

Developing a plan for Lorenzo was slightly different from when Corinna and I faced our cancers. Given that he was a young adult, creativity became a priority. Our intention was to make his time in the hospital as uplifting and positive as possible, both to maximize his chances for recovery, and if he wasn't going to survive, make his remaining time as happy as it could be. My own time in the hospital had been pure isolation and misery, and we wanted to ensure that Lorenzo's experience was very different. During visiting hours there would be ten people in his room. There was so much companionship, so much fun and laughter, that even when Lorenzo had lost thirty pounds and looked like he was wasting away, there was still a smile on his face. When the chemo finally began to affect his hair noticeably, his entire support group took turns shaving their heads in the hospital room. We couldn't have asked for a better group of friends for him.

We did our best to avoid doom and gloom, and we made sure that Lorenzo got up and about instead of staying in bed all day. We had him walking around the halls, and his friends arranged crafts and all sorts of activities. At one point, they ordered a bunch of plastic toy musical instruments, and they formed a band. They'd all play together for a couple of hours and just have a good time. It may sound like a particularly silly activity, but watching Lorenzo experience such joy was beyond compare.

It's true that Lorenzo's treatment was far different from what we'd experienced, both his time in the hospital and in his outpatient procedures. To be sure, that was partly due to medical progress. But it was also due to the way his support team—and there were a lot of us—rallied to his side and kept his days enjoyable. We couldn't get medical advancements on demand, but we could work on controlling his environment. We gave him something to look forward to when he woke up, and we were careful not to press him to do more when he couldn't. I think that made all the difference, especially since his odds of recovery weren't all that encouraging. By luck and effort, what we did worked, and he made it.

I promise to tell you more about my family's experiences with cancer and treatment, but now that you know a little something about us, it's time to put the focus on you.

CHAPTER 3

COMMITTING TO TREATMENT

P robably one of the strangest and most difficult things each of
us—Corinna, Lorenzo, and I—had to do when facing cancer
was to consciously acknowledge our commitment to living.
Especially for Corinna and me, before we could even start
making any plans for how to proceed through the days and weeks,
we each needed to make a commitment to ourselves to put in all
our effort, every step of the way. For us, that meant we needed to
understand something: it didn't matter who we were, what we had
done with our lives to that point, or who we still wanted to become.
Our cancers just came on the scene, and we had to deal with them.
There were not many times that we felt it was unfair for three of the
four of us to experience cancer. We worked on replacing any hints

of self-pity with an awareness of the opportunities to appreciate life each and every day.

I know that some people think of their cancer as a punishment. To me, that seems like a truly harmful thought. No one deserves cancer, and no one should ever be asking themselves what they did to deserve it. We've all seen cancer happen to people who seem to us to have lived healthily and well. And we've all seen cancer happen to people whose habits may have contributed to their getting the disease.

Whatever form of cancer you may be dealing with, it's not going to let you off the hook without a fight, and you're the one who's going to have to do most of the fighting.

My point is this: even if you were a smoker and you got lung cancer, your cancer is not a punishment. It's just basic causality; you were regularly exposed to something that causes cancer. What's harmful about self-blame in light of a cancer diagnosis is that can be a major obstacle to gathering the energy and determination that we need to put toward living.

Whatever form of cancer you may be dealing with, it's not going to let you off the hook without a fight, and you're the one who's going to have to do most of the fighting. What the doctors do is the easy part. They deliver the treatments and wish you the best. With a few exceptions, they don't know what cancer treatment feels like any more than your auto mechanic knows what getting a transmission flush feels like. To choose treatment is to make a commitment to the fight. Taking control of how you approach living through your treatment takes some tough-minded optimism. Being a cancer warrior is not a learned behavior or one passed down through family tradition. Your success will take thoughtful preparation and should include a structured plan for keeping hold of everything you have worked so hard for, including your very life.

Maybe the survival odds they've quoted you aren't great. At the risk of sounding insensitive, I'm going to ask: So what? If a particular form of cancer has a 20 percent survival rate, that's still one person living through it out of five. Why can't you be that one who makes it? If people assumed they'd always lose, no one would ever play the lottery. I don't want to equate playing the lottery with facing cancer treatment, but I do want to point out that we have a funny kind of optimism when it comes to taking a chance in circumstances like the lottery, where the odds are preposterously much worse than the survival rate for any type of cancer. Attitudes like "Hey. Somebody has to win. Why not me?" or "What do I have to lose? A buck?" are not about the odds. They're about *hope*—the hope of winning and getting rich, and the ease of expressing that hope when it comes to games of chance. With cancer, you're hoping to win and keep living. The big difference is that with the lottery there's not much risk; the lottery doesn't require our fortitude or commitment or any hard work on our parts. Expressing hope in that instance is easy. But cancer invites questions about just how much hope you have when it comes to fighting for your life and how willing you are to express it, even to ask other people to join you in feeling it. There are a lot of ways of being insincere about hope up until the moment when a cancer diagnosis comes on the scene. Taking on treatment might be the moment when we first have to ask ourselves—and then prove to ourselves and others—just how much hope we're capable of.

If you're facing cancer treatment, ask yourself, what do you have to lose by giving survival your best shot? Even if you give it your best and don't make it, what might you gain? What is still okay to hope for realistically? Maybe it's visits with grandkids, conversations with friends, or beautiful sunsets, your work, your pets, sitting in the park, eating as many pieces of pie as you like. Whatever it is that makes you glad you woke up and were present any given day, those things are probably still available to you. If you commit to fighting your cancer, you're refusing to be a victim or to think of yourself as a victim— whether of your circumstances or of cruel fortune. Whatever the numbers say, I want to challenge you to believe that you're worth taking a chance on.

There will be people working to help you get through this, but none of that will matter if you don't commit to helping them help you. And that requires you to be brave, even heroic. This may be the biggest challenge you have faced, and you need to find, inside, the energy and determination to move through it. My best sense of things is that that energy comes from believing that you're up for the challenge.

We talk ourselves out of taking on challenges in all sort of ways, and focusing on the risk of discomfort and failure is one way that we rationalize our avoidance. If you never ask someone on a date, you'll never get turned down, but you'll never get that first kiss either. If you never try to run that distance, lift that weight, or climb that hill, you'll never experience the discomfort that must be endured to do those things, and you'll never suffer the embarrassment of finding out it's too far, too heavy, or too steep. You'll also never really know if you could have done it or what it feels like when you succeed. We talk ourselves out of something we want to do or to have, even going so far as to convince ourselves that it's an unworthy or foolish goal. We do it with big, scary things, and we do it with little scary things too: "If I tried to walk across that log, I'd just fall in the water. And if I made it to the other side, so what? I can already see what's over there. It's pointless to try."

The world stands ready to offer us all sorts of rational-sounding reasons to not go through treatment. On occasion, those reasons are fair and truthful. But mostly, they are just rationalizations we take comfort in, in order to save ourselves the trouble of trying and the disappointment and humiliation that might come from being defeated.

Cancer treatment, without question, is hard. My treatment was one of the hardest times of my life, and the only harder time I ever had was watching my wife and son endure it after me. It's going to be hard for you and your loved ones too. Before you can even think about the details of how to get through it, you have to agree to try, and that means giving up any and all of the rationalizations for quitting. You have to commit fully to the fight that is ahead of you and to making the most of this life that you have. And if you're like me or Corinna, you won't just have to make this commitment at the very start of the process. You'll need to remind yourself of it, and you'll even need to renew your determination regularly, because there will be moments that will challenge your hope more than you ever could have imagined at the start of the process.

I want to point out to you one aspect of cancer treatment that people regularly use to rationalize the decision not to go forward with the whole process. Some people are horrified by the cost of treatments and worry that if they do live, they'll be completely broke, unable to live whatever life they've managed to hold on to by surviving. I won't lie to you: treatment is very expensive (unless they've instituted some amazing single-payer nationalized health care system where you live by the time you read this, of course). But let me also ask: What is money for, if not to help us live? We use our money for food, shelter, clothing, and the like, and when we're sick, medicine goes on that list too.

Does a cancer diagnosis mean that to afford your medicines,

your lifestyle might have to change? Probably yes; most of us can't afford otherwise. But think about this alternative. Shortly after my own treatment, a close friend of mine was battling cancer. I won't go into details, but some of the financial decisions he made to save a few bucks changed the entire trajectory of his treatment, and he lost the battle against his cancer. He had the opportunity and the means to choose a better health plan. If he had done so, he would have received the entirety of his treatment instead of delaying it at the point where it needed to be most aggressive.

Unfortunately, my friend's experience is not that unique. In the United States today, there is a serious disconnect between the dialogue about health promotion and the way that insurance puts a price on your life! Imagine if your physical comfort was compromised by another person or group of people who are in a position to make the final call about your worthiness to receive a treatment or medication. This happens every day, and your awareness of the details can change the outcome. There will be times where you should not settle for second best or compromise on a treatment protocol. The more involved you are, the more you can influence the decisions about how your treatment will proceed.

Be on the lookout for those moments when you are making excuses for your fears and other difficult feelings. Recognize these thoughts for what they are, and don't let them keep you out of the fight.

I've seen people with cancer choose to hold on to whatever money they have, saving it for later, for a rainy day, for their retirement. But when you have cancer is precisely when you need to spend the money that you do have on living as best as you can. It *is* the rainy day. So be on the lookout for those moments when you are making excuses for your fears and other difficult feelings. Recognize these thoughts for what they are, and don't let them keep you out of the fight.

* * *

I can't stress this point enough: it really is so important to keep your spirits up if you're going to live through treatment. You need to actually *want* to live—not just to a time beyond your treatment, but during treatment. The challenge, I think, is that most of us plod along in our routines day after day. We are surviving but not really living. That approach isn't going to work for surviving cancer, especially not when your cancer treatment has you feeling three kinds of awful every day. If you want to live through that, you're going to need to be clear about what you're living *for*. I believe that this is truly the first and most important element of any treatment planning you do, and I've put it first for a reason. Without knowing your reasons for living, why bother doing any of the rest?

For some, this will not be an easy task, but you're going to have to identify why you want to be here on earth. Most of our daily habits and routines don't require us to ask that question. In fact, a lot of them keep us from even wondering about what gives us purpose. But I'm asking you to take a bare-bones approach and to be absolutely explicit about why you would like to live. Remember that night I spent alone in the hospital at the edge of my own life, focusing all my energy on breathing in and out? I might have been pushing myself to go on for quite some time before that night, but it was not until then that I really, definitively, felt my own determination to live. I wanted to be with my wife, to raise our boys, to enjoy our hard-won successes. Your identification of your own desire to live may not be as dramatic a moment as mine was—I hope it isn't. Maybe you already know your reason or reasons for living. If not, find your reason, and be sure that it is *yours* and not anyone else's. You have to know what makes living worth *your* while, and you must be honest with yourself about it.

I say to be honest about what you want because sometimes we commit to doing things for the wrong reasons. We say yes to something because it looks good in the short term, other people encourage it, or we just believe that we *should* say yes to it. Then we find ourselves unsatisfied, disappointed. This is true, too, of our thoughts about what we need to give up in order to get by. If your reason for living is to care for your plants, and you give away your plants, you are not helping yourself survive. It's surprising how many things that brighten our hearts and make us glad to get out of bed we think of as unimportant and treat like frivolous extravagances. But without them, we can begin to feel like there's no reason to get out of bed.

I think the differences in people's attitudes about having cancer come down to this: for some people, getting cancer is basically a wake-up call to take stock of where their lives were headed and then reassess their priorities in light of their diagnoses. For them, standing in the shadow of death makes things that used to seem important look like a waste of time and brings other things—even little daily pleasures—to the forefront. Changing their habits reinvigorates their lives, and they work on being happier now than ever before. For others, though, the cancer diagnosis doesn't yield any changes or adjustments to their lives at all, or worse, they choose to let cancer lead their lives rather than take the lead in determining how they will spend whatever time they have. Cancer calls on us to become flexible about life in ways that we might not have considered before.

What we do in response shows us something important about how we choose to live, however many days we have before us still to live.

Identifying why you want to live also means finding ways of keeping that sense of purpose foremost in your mind. It means that you probably need to unhitch yourself from some of your existing beliefs and responsibilities. Whether you live through treatment or not—and especially if you don't—you simply don't have time in your life for junk that you don't want to do but are too embarrassed to opt out of. My suggestion to you is this: put your happiness and your survival first, and get over the awkwardness. Cut the ties that you really don't want in your life anymore. And start believing that you can find enjoyment, even happiness, in each of your days.

I understand that for some people, the pleasure and satisfaction that comes from having many responsibilities might outweigh whatever difficulties arise from maintaining those responsibilities. If you want to live, you'll need to figure out how you can continue to take care of the responsibilities you enjoy, while still, and mainly, taking care of yourself. A real-life example of how *not* to do this well is my buddy Mike. Mike ran a local business when he was diagnosed with stage four colon cancer. That's advanced cancer, and the odds of surviving his particular form of cancer weren't appealing. I called him up to see how he was doing, and he had great news: he was in remission. That *is* great news. That's amazing news. But then I heard some noise on his end of the phone that made me ask him, "Where are you right now?"

He was at work. I laid into him: "What are you doing at work? You're inside a work environment that has contaminants, dust, and all kinds of things that your body doesn't want in front of you right now." He reassured me that he wasn't in the shop but in the office next door. I admitted that this was a little better, but I had to ask him, "Do you *need* to work?" He didn't. He had plenty of money, he told me, and he could leave the day-to-day business in capable hands. "Why are you at work then?" I asked.

"Because," he said, "nobody told me *not* to work."

Nobody told him *not* to. This is what I mean when I say that your doctors are there to kill the thing that's threatening to kill you—but that's all. Your treatments are only one side of the coin. The things I most want to encourage you to focus on are on the other side of that coin. If you don't absolutely *have to* work, don't work during your treatment. When I was going through my own treatment, I didn't feel like I had any choice but to do certain things, like taking those harassing calls from our lender. I *had* to. But I would've been much better off if I could have come up with a way to avoid that. If I'd been able to hand those calls off, my stress level would have been way lower than it was, and my health would have been way better for it.

Maybe you're in a situation in which you don't feel you have any choice but to work. In that case, my advice is to figure out how to do as little as you can. Cancer treatment is a full-time job. If you need to keep working during treatment, find out how to arrange the lightest version of light duty. Don't be shy about trying to arrange your work life in this way. And don't forget that the Family and Medical Leave Act (FMLA) is one of the protections in place that can help you keep your medical coverage while you take a leave of absence from, or cut down on, your work.

You are literally fighting for your life. You need to call in all the benefits to which you're entitled at work, and you'll probably need to distance yourself from some naysaying colleagues in the process. Anybody who can't respect that you need to save your strength for this fight is probably someone who won't be able to care about you more than they care about work going forward. But my question for you is this: Who cares if they think less of you for taking it easy at work or, preferably, taking a temporary leave? Much as we don't like to entertain the thought, we're all only one asset of many that our companies and organizations have at their disposal. Your life, though, is the only one you have. You need to put the needs of your job second (or third, or fourth), so you can hold onto your life.

* * *

I want to share one more thought about what I think it means to really commit to treatment. If I asked you to make a list of the most important people in your life, would you put yourself on that list? My guess is that most people wouldn't. They'd list their spouse, their immediate family, maybe the one brother they like, maybe any living parents, and a couple of close friends. Their own name would never make the list. That's probably the case even after they've added in their least favorite nieces and nephews out of guilt. Most of us weren't raised to feel comfortable putting ourselves on a list of important people, let alone putting ourselves first on that list. But cancer treatment should flip that habit of ours on its head. When you think about what's most important in your life, you need to put yourself (and making the most of your life) on the top of that list. You need to be your own priority.

My personal plan included making a conscious commitment to myself and my survival. That approach was not limited to my treatment but encompassed an overall life plan identifying every area of concern. My suggestion to you is to develop a simple but effective plan for this new phase of your life. In the remaining chapters, l will continue to outline what I strongly believe are the primary components of any plan for your success. These include treatment, behavior, family relationships, personal responsibilities, pain management, and your public persona too. No medical team will address all of these, so you will need to be the one to set yourself a plan and stick to it.

The next most important step after identifying your reasons for living is preparing a stable mind and being present for every moment of your day. That may sound easy to some of you, but the experiences coming your way are going to be new and confusing, and for the most part, they are not going to be either positive or enlightening. How quickly can you digest and mentally deal with terrible news from your doctors? That is going to be one of the hardest tasks you will ever undertake, and not my words or any counselor's words, but your own determination, will be what dramatically impacts how you choose to move forward.

If you haven't yet, I want to invite you to take a moment right now to let out your feelings about your cancer diagnosis, to vent, to get newly pissed off, or to have a big cry. I encourage you to do it now and release that tension from your body. The direction in which we're headed in this book is to find ways of containing all those emotions into small segments of time so that they do not overwhelm your days. Hurt, pain, and suffering need a special moment, but that moment cannot stretch out and interfere with your fight to kick cancer's ass. The plan that I am asking you to formulate should ease your uncertainty, give you stability, and allow you to face with confidence anything that comes your way. Conquering your cancer takes a warrior's approach. If there's a delicate china doll where your warrior needs to be, you are going to have to find a way to bring the warrior to the fore.

CHAPTER 4

CUSTOMIZING YOUR PLAN BASED ON WHAT MATTERS MOST

My approach to cancer is very different from that of any medical professional you will meet. Most of those professionals probably have never fought to save their own lives or created a plan to save two of their closest loved ones. Medical professionals execute their training in a systematic fashion intended to provide a calculated outcome for your symptoms. But what I'm offering here is an account of my real experience digesting and coping with a pile of unorganized, complicated, and usually less-than-positive information, along with my ideas about how to sort that information into various compartments in a way that can bring joy and hope into your life.

After clarifying my reasons for living, my general approach was to design a plan or script—a very flexible script, but a script nonetheless. I felt like all my reasons for living clearly required me to do this as a way of moving forward. I knew I had some choices when it came to the setting, the ways a scene could play out, and who the characters would be. Thinking about my script helped me do two things: focus on an outcome and capture my fellow characters into the process.

You've done your best to clearly identify your reason(s) for living. You've figured out how to let go of obligations that will challenge your ability to focus on treatment and day-to-day living. You've shared your determination with those closest to you and are fully committed to making a go of it. Here's where your script comes into the picture. Assume that you'll have to spend about one hour each day in treatment. Ultimately, the amount of time you spend in treatment will depend on your form of cancer, but an hour a day is a reasonable estimate. You may remember back in chapter 1 where I described the loneliness that can accompany going through the treatment process. Given my and my family's experience, I'm making the assumption that you're going to feel, and maybe actually be, alone a lot. My best advice is to get comfortable with that. One way to adjust is to ask yourself: What am I going to do with the other twenty-three hours each day, all those hours that I am not in treatment? I think that your answer to this question affects not only your chances for your short-term survival but also your happiness in both the short and longer term.

You may say, "But I don't know how I'll feel during those remaining hours of each day," and that's likely very true. How you feel during the course of your treatment can also change dramatically as treatment progresses. But even though there are unpredictable days, weeks, and months to come, and even though it's very important to try to be flexible in your approach to each and every day, I also want to encourage you to plan or script your days to the extent that you can. I think it's important to make a conscious effort to consider at least two things: *what* specifically you choose to do during the time you have, and *whom* you choose to spend that time with. I'm calling the sum of these two main choices your Life Plan.

This may seem like an odd way of putting it, but I think that once you've identified your reasons for living, what's needed next is to plot your future. Let me explain. I'm not talking about plans like buying a house or a car. I'm talking about a future that's bigger and more significant than any one short-term goal. This is a whole different level. You may have never asked yourself what your future should look like in this big and broad sense, but now is precisely the time for full commitment to a vision—your vision, and one that is tailored to give you direction and persistence overall. I'm talking about the future in this way because I think that your overall picture matters when it comes to doing things that might change your day-to-day living for the better. What I'm encouraging you to do here is to plot each of your days according to your vision of how your life should be lived.

Your Life Plan, a daily program that you can live with, needs to be written down. My suggestion is to get a large whiteboard so that you can easily modify your plan as you live it. I am someone who really

> *I think it's important to make a conscious effort to consider at least two things: what specifically you choose to do during the time you have, and whom you choose to spend that time with.*

does not digest rules well, so I only set up one rule that I encourage you to follow: *your Life Plan must contain all positive information.* For example, I reached a point during treatment that on chemo days, when I was anticipating a needle blood draw and a piercing for entry through my port, either the threshold of pain was reduced too low or my anxiety was up too high. The thought of a needle or any procedure involving anything invasive became too much to cope with. My positive approach was to develop a personal plan to control anxiety and take my mind off the task. I could not entirely control the pain and discomfort, but I could make a simple alteration like bringing my headphones and a favorite playlist to distract my thoughts. At home, my favorites were Ozzy Osbourne's "Crazy Train," or AC/DC's "Highway to Hell," and on a really good day, Run-DMC's "Hard Times," but to relax during chemo treatment, I strongly preferred classical.

If you take the time daily to structure and adjust your plan, your growing resilience will help you overcome both fears and disappointments along the way.

On any given day, the extent to which you are in touch with your Life Plan is likely to vary, but having the awareness to create (and recreate) that plan will change the outcome of your experience for the better. As you think about what's important at this point in your life, you might even be surprised to notice that you challenge yourself at a level higher than you've ever done before. You'll also build resilience as you move toward your goals and take more and more decisive, positive actions. If you take the time daily to structure and adjust your plan, your growing resilience will help you overcome both fears and disappointments along the way.

I usually tell folks to begin by removing all expectations. Most people freak when I describe what I mean: if we remove all expectations, there will be no disappointment. "But how?" people ask. In place of the expectations, we are developing and executing a personal plan for your success. It's definitely not a simple thing to do, but it also gets easier with daily practice and attention to your behavior patterns, especially those that arise when your expectations are not met. Following a plan can actually help you remove expectations and help you digest whatever outcomes come your way.

Here's one example. During my hospital visits, I began to experience a lack of rest and even nightly insomnia. As you might imagine, this did not help with recovery. At the time, I tried to examine why, but I did not fully understand why I was suffering from lack of sleep until years later. What I *was* able to notice were little details about my time in the hospital that I could try to change. I realized that being close to the nurses' station made my insomnia and restlessness worse. The constant activity and noise kept me hypervigilant; to this day, lots of activity nearby not only keeps me from relaxing but actually agitates my distress. I believed that repositioning my room location could change the outcome of my stay, and so on one visit, I made a big request to the head nurse to avoid that particular location. Just making the request and speaking up about my needs felt like I was contributing to my well-being. And it worked! From then on, I requested a room location at the beginning of each hospital stay. There was no disappointment with further hospital visits. I had used awareness of my needs and polite and effective communication to eliminate a clear source of disappointment.

There are reasonable requests you can make within each facet of your Life Plan. The needs that arise for you during treatment may be brand new to you. You may never have said them out loud, and you may never even have thought about them until they pop up during your treatment. That is why now is precisely the right time to design a plan to meet those needs and to track that plan by keeping a record of your development. Even a seemingly little thing, like the simple habit of picking up a Starbucks coffee in the morning, does not need to be eliminated if you are unable to leave the house. Figure out how to make it work. Plan it through, buy the grounds or beans, and make a cup at home. Eliminate disappointment, focus on the positive, and control the outcomes that are still in your hands.

During the early part of my treatment, I started to notice that my day was dominated by boredom. I was going mad from the repetitiousness of my experiences as a cancer patient. The combination of no productivity and loss of freedom was a kick in the ribs; it challenged my very sense of integrity and went against my belief in myself as a productive and active person who contributes to the world. "What the hell am I going to do now in this condition?" was my constant question to myself. As a cancer patient, there wasn't much I could contribute to my family, our business, or our community. That major obstacle of feeling confined and immobilized actually played a role in motivating me to develop a personal plan. For me, structuring my Life Plan was all about making a constant movement in an upward direction. In a sense, that meant turning my cancer diagnosis and treatment into a useful tool to change my life. On the one hand, I realized that this was a period of my life in which I needed to be a "taker" rather than a contributor. On the other hand, I wanted to find ways to feel like I could still contribute, given my limitations.

* * *

In our family, each one of our Life Plans was unique. There were common themes, but the choices and individual scripts were very different. Though I did not know to expect it at the time, the number of responsibilities and complications in my own plan ended up providing me with a foundation to help guide Corinna and then Lorenzo through theirs. Observations from my own cancer experience became relevant when Corinna and Lorenzo each experienced similar phases of their cancer processes. What was the same for each of us was our attempts to live each day's uncertainty by thinking of it within the context of where our lives were headed and how we intended to get there. We each had to do that in the face of numerous and mounting worries.

I'd always considered myself to be forward thinking or future oriented; dwelling on and reliving the past was never a practice of mine. So for me, a major source of worry was the constant unknown conditions of my own treatment. My objective was survival, but the absence for so long of any decisive prognosis inflamed my wandering mind and led me to dwell on all the possibilities for what was yet to come. It was a new task I was eager to master, but there was no *Cancer Survival for Dummies* book for me to follow. To help stir up my worries was that cocktail of mind-altering pain medication I mentioned before. It was a perfect storm: a foggy mind plagued by worries about the future. There was no Aladdin's lamp for me to wish on. In a very real sense, I had to wrestle with my worry head on so that I could regain a sense of freedom in my daily life. The appreciation of mobility was what I held on to, and I let that appreciation motivate my desire to climb back to a level of everyday living where I had more and more physical freedom. I wanted to gain back my ability to have my movements be pain free. The only restrictions I wanted to grapple with were the ones that were imposed by me. I was sure of one thing: fear that my cancer was a death sentence was not going to have a place in my plan.

Each day came to feel special because I wanted to improve my own situation and be able to pass those improvements along to others who faced similar situations. Imagine how strange it felt when Corinna was the next person in my life to have cancer. I was already motivated to share what I'd practiced and learned through my experience, but passing along to her my idea about designing a Life Plan was, well, a bit choppy. What had worked for me wasn't going to be identical for her, so there was some experimenting that she had to do herself in order to find her way.

One thing that did work for us both, though, was that I could take the ideas I'd formed while going through treatment and make them the focus of my experience as a caregiver for Corinna. From the first phone call when Corinna shared with me her diagnosis, I began to perform a strategy for her Life Plan without her even being an informed part of it. The only thing I could be at that moment was a mentor committed daily to supporting her success. We both already knew that Corinna had a tendency to worry and that her tendency could evolve in any number of directions, each of which would take her mind to an unpleasant or even dark place. My new job as a caregiver was to keep Corinna looking forward in a positive direction and to eliminate as many unknown conditions as possible so that she would have a sense of stability during each day.

That meant having to be creative. There are surprisingly few choices for a patient during treatment. If you're claustrophobic but need an MRI to determine the presence of a cancerous growth, you have no choice but to enter the chamber and lie still until the procedure is finished. I recently experienced my own worst performance during an MRI on my shoulder. After a dozen or so MRIs so far in my lifetime, this most recent one was the one that broke me. I was prepared and feeling good, understanding I needed to be motionless for twenty minutes. It was cold in the room, so I requested a warm blanket for comfort. As the tray rolled my body into the tunnel, I noticed that this particular machine at the VA was some ancient relic; I felt stuffed into a space much smaller than any machine I'd experienced before. After only thirty seconds, I squeezed the ball and elected to stop the procedure. Wow—for the first time, I'd failed my MRI! I was well aware that my shoulder had extensive pain and that completing the MRI was necessary for a diagnosis. I had to find my inner warrior, place my shoulder back into the harness for twenty minutes, and endure the pain. On the second try, I completed the MRI, and the doctors were able to diagnose a partial tear to my right rotator cuff.

For many of the tests you may need to undergo, you may never know what you are about to do unless you ask exactly what the entire experience entails. And even if you were given some explanation, there may still be other aspects of the test or procedure that you were not warned about beforehand. Most medical procedures remain mysterious to most of us until we go through them. Explanations tend to be limited at best; if there is time beforehand, you may receive a pamphlet to satisfy your curiosity, but that's about it. But that doesn't mean that you don't have alternatives. With an MRI, for example, there may be more than one kind of machine at your testing site—ones that are more open or even allow you to sit up and watch television! And if you must lie in the chamber, you should talk to your tech about options: covering your eyes with a towel, having a blanket over your torso for comfort, listening to music, bringing a friend into the room with you, taking a sedative, practicing meditative breathing.

I wanted to do everything in my power to prepare Corinna for all the mystery and to remove as much of that mystery as I possibly could. To the best of my ability, I could not live up to that promise. The mental preparation for each individual experience was epic, and not epic as in "memorable" or as in "Damn, I want to experience this again!" These epic experiences are the ones you want to put into a closet, close the door tight, and then also nail it permanently shut. I've come to identify unknown surprises as scars—not physical scars, of course, but scars that sit deep in your mind. Unfortunately, there are experiences you may need to go through for the sake of survival, and they include poking, probing, and sometimes also pain that you never thought possible.

I knew from my experience that even as prepared as you may be, some surprises and deviations from the plan will still occur. As systematically as some treatment plans might be laid out, there will still be the issue of having to cope with modifications as well as changes to your own body along the way. Corinna and I worked on approaching treatment with flexibility, loosening up our expectations so that we could adapt to whatever changes came along. We both felt that treatment was extremely experimental; as professional as the medical staff appeared, they really seemed to us to be winging it all the time. The more flexible we were able to be, the more we reduced our chances of disappointment at each step along the way.

The same was true for Lorenzo. As any child might be, Lorenzo was a delicate, fragile soul during treatment. And it was a challenge for me to reassure him by saying "everything is going to be all right" when I knew we couldn't say that with any certainty. The first reaction as a parent is usually a bit selfish, an indulgence of parental feelings, sometimes with little consideration for the feelings of your child. I, for one, found it difficult to pull myself together and wear my game face during the entirety of Lorenzo's treatment process. It was hard for me to gauge what to do or figure out how best to comfort my son while standing by his side during the lowest point of his young life. The one benefit we did have during Lorenzo's treatment was that the medical staff and the treatment plan were structured with little room for error. That there was a clear path for his treatment meant the elimination of any confusion on our parts about next steps. Because that was so different from either my or Corinna's experience, it gave the entire family an opportunity to attend to Lorenzo's Life Plan with more detail and consideration than during our two previous experiences.

The entire family wanted to make his shitty journey less dreary, and so we worked together to see a brighter side of life and include uplifting experiences whenever it was appropriate. This is where our family's journey through cancer really changed. It took two prior goes at it, both with a less-than-enjoyable lifestyle, but with Lorenzo, we found a way to overcome the obstacles and turn a seeming death sentence into a fun factor. The setting for our fun would change weekly—from the hospital to our house—but one thing was certain: if you were to join in Lorenzo's Life Plan, there was no room for your tears. Lorenzo's personal plan clearly identified one guiding idea: this battle was not going to suck the life out of him. We decided to be as creative as we could in finding ways to celebrate our bond. I remember one occasion, after Lorenzo's chemo treatment and before his bone marrow transplant, when he spent about a month at home. He really wanted to go to a rave that was happening just outside of town. Corinna and I bought VIP-area passes for the four of us, and when Lorenzo put on his face mask before going into the club, so did Corinna, Dominic, and I. As a family, we went in and enjoyed the rave, all four of us looking like we'd dressed up as cancer patients. We had a blast, and Lorenzo got to enjoy the music and even some dancing, just like he would have were he not also an actual cancer patient. The result of our efforts to be creative was that our family at this point in time felt really confident. That feeling was a wonderful surprise; we had regained an entire emotion that had been taken away from our young family for years. Of course, not every day was abundant, but the ones that were had been designed to give us all a sense of having epic fun and great memories that could balance out the slog of Lorenzo's cancer battle. Each member of the family listened to Lorenzo's thoughts and helped put his ideas into action.

* * *

In the rest of this chapter, I want to give you a few things to think about as you design and modify your Life Plan. The first of these is to become a master of paying attention to your body.

Throughout treatment, your body will be your everyday point of focus. You will need to get in tune with it or start being present in it in a way that might feel brand new and more important to you than before. Consider doing things like taking a deep breath and appreciating the preciousness of the ability to breathe, stretching your limbs and feeling the pleasure of that tension and release. There may come a day when you can't take these things for granted anymore. You may find your lungs so filled with fluid that your breathing sounds like a pot of boiling water. The day may come when your idea of exercise is using a spirometer to check your lung volume.

I've already asked you to identify what motivates you to keep breathing when it's not easy anymore. Every day is a chance to reaffirm your answer or find what gives you that motivation. Life *will* be different from what it was before, and your body is likely to demand your attention in ways you're not used to, but you can still face each day on your terms. To do that, you will have to move beyond merely following the paths and instructions offered by your team of professionals who only know you by your patient chart. Since your medical team is going to be entirely focused on your body in one particular way, your task is to focus on it by tuning in to everything it is telling you.

I really believe that thinking about the basic elements of your everyday health is very closely related to thinking about your happiness. When we're sick, feeling sluggish, or simply have a headache, it's a lot harder to be present, emotionally steady, and upbeat. If you're in pain, you're less patient with yourself and other people. If the pain lingers for a few days, it's normal to start wondering if it's worth the discomfort to even wake up for the next one. That's exactly the experience we're looking to head off. So I'm asking you to focus on your body so that you can feel as good as possible throughout treatment and beyond.

Paying attention to your body involves examining the way you spend your time and energy. Too many of us are stuck in a familiar rut. We repeat behaviors and physical routines day after day that we don't even notice or that we didn't even choose for ourselves. We just took the path of least resistance, and over time, it stuck. In other words, we're living and moving around on autopilot. Have you ever been heading to work or maybe the grocery store when you suddenly look around and wonder where you are or can't quite remember how you got there? You navigate to these places and through your days largely by habit. What happens when you first get home after work? Maybe you walk your dogs. Or you might head right into the shower to wash the day away. On any given day, you're capable of doing any variety of things when you come in the door, but chances are good that you'll do what you usually do. That isn't necessarily bad, but depending on the habits you've cultivated, it could become a problem during treatment. To get through cancer treatment, take inventory of your physical habits, and start weeding out the ones that aren't helping you survive or thrive.

* * *

Along with paying attention to your body's signals comes taking care with what you put into your body. Whatever your habits have been, this is the time to take a big step back and remember, or learn, how to eat.

Chemo and some radiation therapies are likely to destroy your appetite. You may experience mouth sores or a dulling of your sense of taste. In my own experience, ordinarily flavorful foods like pizza and burgers tasted bland. The things you've normally enjoyed eating might not seem appealing. But you'll need to keep fueling your body, despite getting less pleasure from food. If you are lucky enough to avoid mouth sores and can have solid food, your plan will be easier. You might be asked to go on a neutropenic diet, which can help fortify your weakened immune system. No matter what, in order to protect yourself from what are otherwise some pretty normal bacteria, you'll need to make sure to cook foods completely so that all bacteria are destroyed. There are probably going to be easier days, and then more difficult days, when it comes to eating and nutrition. If you can think of food as fuel during this time, you'll do well. You want to focus on putting the best—and best-prepared—fuel into your body. That means avoiding a Snickers candy bar diet, with the one exception that you should indulge in that Snickers if it's the only appetizing thing that you can find.

During one of my hospital stays, the staff physician noted that I was losing two pounds a day. I had mouth sores and was taking in less than one thousand calories a day on my neutropenic diet, and my immune system was failing. I had reached the point where the nurses secured my room, and all visitors were required to wear protective suits in order to come in. No outside food was allowed in, the hospital food choices were limited, and I found them all completely undesirable. On his daily visit, the doctor laid out my options: if I could not exceed two thousand calories on my own within two days' time, he would have no choice but to insert a feeding tube into my throat. That was a "No way!" moment for me, so I quickly came to understand that staying alive meant that I had the task of forcing a realistic nutrition plan quickly into place. I'm asking you to take an honest look at your habits and choose in favor of a good result from treatment.

* * *

The next area of focus is your bodily movement and activity. Having an active lifestyle was my normal day, and accepting a sedentary lifestyle was a new experience for me. It was part of my practice to believe that a little exercise lifts your mood and helps you stay positive. When I was in the hospital, I kept as active as I could. Plenty of days, all I could do was rest, so that's what I did. But moving around made all the difference. If I had the energy to get up and walk the halls, I seized the opportunity. If I had a little spring in my step, I'd go climb some stairs. Some days, I even asked the physical therapist to bring an exercise bike to my room. There were several days when I coached Lorenzo on an hourly basis to get out bed and walk the hospital halls and to create a habit of wandering around different floors or walking to the elevator visit the courtyard downstairs. Reluctantly, and with some pain or frustration, Lorenzo came to understand deeply the positive power of physical movement during treatment.

Day by day, do what you can to *safely* be active. Your medical team can help determine what's right for you, so ask them what level of activity is okay and what is best for your current phase of treatment. Everybody works at different fitness levels, so there is no need to compare yourself to anybody else. You'll also want to keep in mind that nobody in treatment is capable of doing what he or she could before cancer. Do what you can do each day. Even if it's opting to walk down the hallway, I promise you'll feel better than you would if you just sat in bed all the while.

Anything that's possible, any physical movement that you can achieve, be sure to record it and then duplicate it. You can make changes *today* to improve both your emotional state and how you feel physically by moving your body. Please take advantage of the opportunities available to you to eat and drink better and to move your body when, and to the extent that, you can. You'll better your chances for a happier life both during and on the other side of treatment.

* * *

The fourth area of focus is on your emotions, especially when it comes to the business of reducing negative emotions like stress, anger, jealousy, and resentment. The source of these emotions doesn't really matter, from being pissed off at a family member's thoughtless comment to getting steamed by politics on TV. Anything that makes your blood boil or gets your thinking obsessively counts as stress inducing. *Stress feeds the cancer* and not your health. You'd be smart to step away from things you know to be stress inducing for you. Don't complicate your illness because you have a habit of arguing on the internet or being upset with your boss or your neighbor.

The important thing is to acknowledge the presence of our negative emotions and then put some effort into setting them aside before they land us in worse health. I know it's possible to feel helpless in relation to your worst inclinations. But I'm telling you that the better the job you do avoiding stressors during your treatment, the more control you will feel you have, and the more you will know that your own efforts during this process are the best they could be. My point here (it is small but, I hope, useful) is to focus on retraining your negative emotions so that even when facing fear and instability and all the challenges that come your way, you can achieve a kind of centeredness in your overall approach.

Inventory what you know to be your own negative habits involving your attitudes and feelings. What are the specific things always going on in your mind or your feelings that do not contribute positively to your well-being in the long term or that will ultimately make you less capable of experiencing and enjoying life? These are the things you'll want to work on. The more of them you can decrease or redirect into more productive thoughts or activities, the better each day will become.

Most of the news I received during cancer treatment was lousy, and I struggled to cope with each new detail. So I worked on preparing myself by acknowledging that sometimes during treatment, I would get bad news. It could be that my cancer wasn't responding to the therapy or that I would need to extend treatment. Whatever that news was, it was hard at first not to let it ruin my day. The way I approached my feelings was like this: I was going to feel what I was going to feel, and I needed to be honest about that. I didn't want to put on a fake smile and stuff down those feelings under cover of false positivity. I wanted actually to *be* more positive. A simple strategy that helped me was to isolate the negative emotions into a small, contained portion of my day. This took practice. It is most definitely not a discipline that came easily for me. Sometimes I even set a timer. Once I got better at containment, the time I gave the bad feelings grew shorter. I would do my best to work through the bad news and give it its space and then not let it bleed into the rest of my day. Eventually I could contain my negative emotions into smaller and smaller segments of the day, which left me more time for enjoying life.

* * *

At the same time that you inventory and watch out for your negative habits, be sure to make a list of positive feelings and things you like to do. Ideally, you're going to pinpoint the things in life that truly motivate you to live (and not the things that serve as temporary solutions or Band-Aids to your pains). What makes you laugh, sing, or dance around the kitchen when nobody's looking? Think about these positive things as you prepare for treatment, and think about them during treatment too, because they may change as you go through that process. If doing something makes you glad you woke up in the morning, write it down. It can be a chat with a loved one or a devotional practice. Look for the simple things that you appreciate. What you pick doesn't have to sound amazing or even interesting to anybody else. If watching a cooking show and trying to recreate a recipe sounds like a good time to you, put it on the list. There can be little things in your daily plan that can really improve your mood; for me, that was telling people that I loved them and asking for their patience when I needed it.

People don't like talking about dying, but not having our end in focus can keep us from really living today. So create that list of the things that make you glad you're alive. Those are the things you need to build into habits. Some of them probably are part of your habit already, but most of us can do more than we do to bring these things to the forefront of our everyday lives.

Once you have your list, try swapping out a negative habit for a more positive one: substitute a daily practice of something that you find uplifting for a habit that brings you down, or just give more time to the positive experiences (including any new ones you discover) as you work on eliminating the less positive ones. If you have a routine that leaves you feeling isolated, cultivate a new habit that gets you interacting with people. Maybe your situation is the opposite of that, and you need to carve out part of your day to do something entirely alone. Whatever charges your batteries, do that instead of the things that drain you.

* * *

I've pointed out that you're not likely to have a whole lot of "good days" during treatment—days when you're feeling vibrant and alive both mentally and physically. If you find that you only feel that way once a week, obviously, you won't be able to pack everything you'd like to do that week into that one good day. But if you approach things systematically, you can make the most of each good day you get.

Chemo days, for example, might be relatively good days for you. Granted, there is the discomfort of the infusion itself, potential bloating from the saline, or common complications like an infected port, the nurse missing a vein during a blood draw, tender skin, or a rash. But we already know that if you're prepared going in for what could happen and pay attention to how your body reacts to your treatment, then when something does go wrong, there's likely to be less confusion and a quicker path to resolution of the problem. And if your chemo treatment goes smoothly, maybe that's a day you'll take the opportunity to do something nice for yourself. Catch a movie on the way home from the clinic, or fit in a fun outing to buoy your spirits. The memory of the good time you had can help you smile later in the week when you might be feeling lousy. It'll remind you that life's not all suffering.

Take your lists and get to work trying to find the good in every day. Cultivating good habits and a positive attitude will go a long way to helping you get through hard days. I've met a few people who are such champions of positivity that even their hard days are still good days. That's a tall order, but every step you take toward that goal is going to result in a happier you, whatever your day brings. And if you practice it enough, having a positive attitude will become your habit. Getting better and trying to have a little joy in your day—these constitute your full-time job. The better you do that job, the better your chances of getting back to taking care of all of those other things you care about. You're not likely to have a lot of energy during treatment. Invest what energy you do have in sustaining and finding pleasure in your own life.

The people who love you actually *need* you to focus on your happiness, insofar as that's what makes you capable of being present with them. Unfortunately, they won't always understand that. Some of them won't comprehend why you can't keep up with the things you used to do. Others may overwhelm you with attempts to be helpful. In the next chapter, we'll talk about what you can do to communicate positively with those around you on behalf of finding satisfaction in your day-to-day life.

CHAPTER 5

LEADING YOUR TEAM BY COMMUNICATING CLEARLY

The night we were told our son Lorenzo had leukemia, we reached out to a core group of people who were important in Lorenzo's life and in ours. By the time some of them arrived at the hospital, Dr. Abbas had administered Lorenzo's symptom-relief cocktail, and Lorenzo was up and walking around the room. At that moment, our friends looked to be in worse shape than he was, and Corinna found herself consoling some of them. I remember thinking that for the mother of a kid who had looked like he was dying just an hour earlier, this was a bizarre position for her to be in.

Our close friends' reactions were pretty common. We aren't

alone in this world, and weird as it may seem to say, we need to remember that most during cancer treatment. When a person is diagnosed with cancer, it sends out shockwaves through his or her entire social network. Corinna described it as a meteorite hitting a house in the middle of town. The person whose house is hit is the most impacted, but the effects don't stop there. The next-door neighbors will take serious losses from debris and fire. The whole neighborhood will be damaged, and people for miles around will be unsettled. They'll keep thinking that it could have been them and that it very nearly was.

We aren't alone in this world, and weird as it may seem to say, we need to remember that most during cancer treatment.

Think about your own cancer diagnosis and the shockwaves that spread out from the impact. Even the people you only know in passing will probably be shaken. Those waves reverberate through your entire social network, but of course they hit those closest to you the hardest. Your loved ones especially will be scared. Sometimes our loved ones can be more afraid than those of us who are actually cancer patients. A cancer diagnosis just reminds everyone of what they are trying to forget: rich or poor, young or old, our lives could be threatened at any time.

* * *

I wish I'd known ahead of time that the reminder of death's nearness was going to affect how people looked at me for quite a while. Friends, family, and coworkers didn't always know how to act around me. That's why I felt that I needed to be deliberate in setting the tone myself. First and foremost, I needed to be the one to stay positive and to let the people around me know that I was making and executing a plan that I had tailored just for me. I wanted them to hear *from me* that I was working on making it through my treatment.

Back in chapter 1, I mentioned how rumors about my illness got started in our neighborhood and eventually lead to Lorenzo and Dominic being bullied at school. It's having experienced that particular consequence of not managing the messaging around my cancer that leads me to make this recommendation to you: in order to take charge of the way people interact with you, you'll need to act fast. Think about that meteorite hitting your house. It's going to start a fire, and that fire will spread. How quickly you get that fire under control is going to determine how much damage it does. The longer you wait to act (or the more you believe that you don't need to act), the worse the response will become. It can be surprising how quickly saving and rebuilding relationships can come to seem impossible. I didn't think to anticipate that happening, so I didn't initially do anything proactive to control the perception of my illness in the neighborhood. Controlling your public story or face can feel like extra work when you're already feeling physically and emotionally overloaded. But to the extent that you can direct that story, the less you will be distressed by other people's responses to you, and the more chances you will have for making the most of them.

This applies to all your relationships, personal, professional, and everything in between. I hope you'll take my advice to take control of public messaging quickly. People seek out news to find out what's happening. If that news isn't coming from you, somebody else will start speculating. The rumor mill is always running, and if people don't know better, they'll listen to whatever's coming out of it. Don't let false information be what your network hears. Likewise, don't let those who are important to you receive thirdhand information that could well distort the truth of your situation or make them feel distant from you. I don't think you should be consumed by what other people think; but I am very aware of the negative health effects *for you* if you don't take other people's curiosity and news-spreading tendencies into consideration. Controlling communications around your cancer is a direct way of taking care of yourself. This is part of your role as a cancer warrior, and it can help you have a decent experience if you plan it out from the beginning.

I could have been resentful of having to be responsible for how others reacted to my illness, and for a little while there, I was. But then I made a firm decision to take charge of what was being communicated in the news broadcast about me! I came to realize that there were at least two aspects of every communication that I had to manage. First of all, I did not want to tell everyone in the world my problems. Maybe you feel the same; there could be any number of reasons for withholding information about your illness. Although I had a pretty unique rationale for keeping my secret from my bank, simply being a private person would have been enough of a reason for me. I wanted to keep unpleasant details about my treatment on a need-to-know basis, even for the people closest to me.

Second, I did not want to be seen as sickly or pitiable. Most of us work all our lives to project an image of competency and confidence. Even if we're sick, we still want to be viewed as accomplished, even admirable. What I want to tell you is that it *can* be that way, but it's going to be up to *you* to make that happen. Now don't go adjusting your other twenty-three hours a day just to look more inspirational! It's okay to limit your concern for everyone else to keeping a smile on your face in social situations. It's not easy to be upbeat when you're not feeling well. If you've done the work of deciding on your public face and making sure that it's not too far removed from your private face, you'll have a far better success rate than someone who hasn't taken those preventative steps. My point is this: be conscious of how you're presenting yourself to the people who witness, or are part of, your life during treatment. That includes not just the people you know but also sometimes complete strangers.

The exciting thing, I think, is that you have all these opportunities to show the world in general that your overall attitude is a positive one. In chapter 4, we worked on making sure that your Life Plan was filled only with positive things. Here, we're just extending that to include how you communicate with everyone around you. I feel that the choices I made about how to think and to behave made a huge difference in my treatment results and continue to make a huge difference in my life posttreatment. I didn't want to do myself any more harm than my cancer was already doing, and I knew the people around me were worried and scared. I wanted to communicate with them in a way that would make them feel at least okay, if not good, about the time they spent with me. I don't think it would be noble to explain cancer as a good thing or something to be proud of, but I do want to emphasize that it certainly is not something to be ashamed of. Communicating constructively means holding your head high and maintaining a positive persona.

* * *

Controlling who knows what about your situation is only half of the puzzle. There's another side of managing the flow of information: make sure that anyone you need as part of your immediate support system gets all the relevant information to be able to support you well. While they certainly don't need to be bombarded with a real-time account of every discomfort you're feeling, there are things you'll be wise to include them in. For example, make very sure the people you need are up to date about simple things like your treatment process, your medicines, and your overall health status. Make even more sure that those same people know *precisely what you need from each of them.*

You'll remember that I wasn't particularly good at this myself. Although we had valid reasons for secrecy, it's pretty clear in retrospect that I took it a little too far by disengaging from some of the supports that I needed. I isolated myself socially at a time when I was already often being isolated physically because of my reduced ability to fight off disease. I should have let more of my inner circle in—the people I really needed on my side so that I could cope with everything that was happening. I needed my team more than I let them be there for me. Partly it was out of legitimate fear of losing our business, but it was mostly out of embarrassment about the condition I was in.

We all need the help of other people to keep us going. Whoever it is—parents, siblings, friends, spouses, spiritual advisors—if you're undergoing treatment, you need to have your support network in place. Some members of your circle of family and friends are closer to the center than others. Make an honest assessment of which people in your life you can really count on when you need them. These are going to be your star players. You'll depend on this all-star team to help you every step along the way. Do you remember back in grade school when you had to pick teams for sports? When you're putting together your support team for treatment, you're the captain. Just like at school, some of the people will be hoping you'll pick them for your team, and certain others will be praying that you won't. Your life depends on these people, so think hard about who will make the best teammates. Who are your top picks, the ones you know will be there for you—the people you feel you can't do this without? Identify your star players, and recruit them quickly. Some people will surprise you along the way, either with their willingness to help or their resistance to being helpful. So this primary group may change a bit, but it's not likely to change dramatically during your treatment.

It's also the case that not everyone in your circle of family and friends is going to make the cut. Maybe you love your aunt, but every time she says she'll be over later, something comes up. You can't afford to depend on her for rides to treatment, so consider not picking her for that role. Maybe one of your friends is a great guy and you two always have a ton of laughs together, but you know he's not particularly good at managing his finances. You're not going to put him in charge of making sure that your bills are paid on time. Your aunt and your friend may be great people to have visit you when you're feeling well enough for social time, but they might be poor choices for your core team.

Of course, you don't want to hurt the feelings of loved ones who offer to help. There may be good reasons that you don't think of them as members of your core team, but there are equally good reasons they're part of your life. If they ask why you aren't leaning on them more for help, let them know your reasoning. Be as gentle and diplomatic in your language as you can, though. They love you, and you don't want to hurt them. You also don't want to miss appointments, mortgage payments, or meals they were supposed to be bringing you just because you couldn't be honest with them. Kindly let them know that you have that other stuff covered, but what they *can* do for you is visit you when you're up for it. They can send you email messages, texts, or cards or even do something specific that you feel comfortable asking them to do. Maintaining your social contact with them can be a great comfort.

* * *

You already know that I struggled with being a "taker" instead of a "giver" during treatment. I had to let the people in my social circle know not to expect me to write back immediately or be available for a visit on any given day. I needed to help them understand that they really couldn't expect much from me. In fact, anything I was able to do with or for someone else was a bonus! My guess is that you, too, will want to keep in touch with family and friends, but you may not be able to do so a lot of the time. You just won't have the energy or feel well enough. The less people expect from you during this time, the less pressure you'll feel to make your day about someone else's happiness or satisfaction. If you're someone who needs permission to release yourself from pressure, I officially give you permission not to give a shit about anyone except yourself. Don't think about it as abusing your health status or, as some people say, "playing the cancer card." Now is the time to point out to others the limitations presented by your cancer. If you give it a chance, you will be surprised how accommodating people will be when you explain to them what you need.

It's even a good idea to manage (or ask one of your core supporters to manage) the people who want to pay you a visit. If you don't, you can be lying in a hospital bed for several days without seeing anybody. Then, everyone will show up on the same day. Multiple groups of people visiting, one after another, won't cheer you up or entertain you. Excess company when you're not feeling well can easily become a burden and leave you feeling exhausted and overwhelmed. People will want to express their concern, to see you and connect with you. And you'll be glad for their visits most of the time. Some days, though, the timing will be bad; particular times of day may be rough too. For me, I needed to be careful about evening time; people were off work and wanted to visit, but this was hands-down my weakest time of the day. There are just going to be moments when your smile slips, and you can't project the positivity that you want to show your visitors.

To manage visits, you could have an email list and send out a little newsletter or weekly update. You could give one of your closest support people the task of sharing information and scheduling visits. If you went with that option, you'd only have to tell that one person, "I'm just not up for visitors today." Then, he or she would be able to call off a visit and reschedule it for another time. This saves you the embarrassment of having to turn someone away. It will be a lot easier for your friend to say you aren't up for a visit than it will be for you to battle any guilt associated with telling someone yourself.

Consider setting up (or having someone set up) a private-message group on social media or use a website that provides a free portal for the sole purpose of keeping family and friends informed during health crises. Lorenzo took the social media message-group option, and it worked great for him. It let people know things like when visits were welcome and when he just wasn't up for it. All he had to do was write, "I'm having a bad day. Please don't come by." The social media option also gives you an easy platform to disseminate news about details that can change week to week. And a private group gives you control over who receives the messages, which is nice if you don't want things broadcast to a wide audience.

There are, of course, far older, time-honored social networks. Maybe you belong to a church group, or a lodge like the Masons or Elks. I'm a member of the Veterans of Foreign Wars. Many times, when I've gone to dinner with the guys, someone will make an announcement. They'll let everyone know that a member is in the hospital or at home recovering from surgery. All the important information is there, such as whether he or she can or can't have visitors right now and so forth. Most importantly, people won't be wondering and worrying about why that member didn't show up for a few weeks.

Whatever methods you decide on to keep your people informed, there are certain things they'll need to know. For instance, the things that are and are not okay for you to be around during your current phase of treatment can vary. At some stages, for example, you're not necessarily going to be able to be near flowers. You'll feel awful if someone shows up with a big, expensive bouquet and you have to explain that you need it to be removed from your room. By the same token, warning people not to wear perfumes or heavy scents around you before they visit will be much better than shooing them out when they arrive. Good communication of your needs is going to be a great way to avoid awkward or hurtful interactions. The fact that people are visiting is thoughtful. You can keep the visits pleasant and beneficial to your well-being by nipping problems like these in the bud, instead of dealing with the fallout afterward.

Dietary restrictions fall into this same category of things to mention to your social circle. *After* someone has bought you a fruit basket or something from your favorite bakery isn't a great time to tell him or her that you can't eat any of it. If you're on a neutropenic diet because your weakened immune system can't handle certain foods, that means Granny's homemade treats would almost certainly be a terrible idea for you. It's better if your circle knows up front that you can't have it. That will also help you avoid the "What could it hurt to have just one?" argument and eating something that can make you uncomfortable or even set back your health and recovery. Head off the problem by being clear about your dietary restrictions as they occur.

Another thing we found that visiting friends and family needed to be prepared for was how different we were going to look to them. If you've lost twenty or thirty pounds, it will come as less of a shock if they've been told beforehand. If you've lost your hair, or shaved it preemptively, let visitors know that too. I remember a visit from a friend when I was extremely bloated from an allergic reaction. My body was so engorged with fluid that I could not fit shoes on my Shrek-looking feet. I hadn't warned him beforehand, and so most of the visit was spent explaining to my friend why my appearance had morphed me into a cartoon character and describing the pain associated with it. Anything that significantly alters the way you look is likely to frighten visitors when they come through the door, and you won't enjoy the look on their faces when they first see you. Prepare them for the changes in your appearance before they arrive so that they have less of a reaction. You'll start the visit on better footing that way, and you'll enjoy yourselves more.

* * *

Naturally, keeping your lines of communication open doesn't begin or end with visitors. Whomever you live with is going to need to know, day to day, how you are doing. You'll need to be aware of days that are taking a turn for the worse and communicate that. It isn't so simple as saying, "Don't come to visit me today." The people around you will need to know what's going on with you more frequently and sometimes in greater detail.

I've seen some people keep a whiteboard on the wall as a mood indicator with either a smiley face or a frown on it. That way, they can display to everybody in the house how they're feeling without saying a word. Not having to repeat over and over that today is rough could prevent some snapping at loved ones who were simply trying to go about their days. You could also add boxes to tick for nausea or other symptoms you might be experiencing. Then family will know to be extra mindful of not making things harder for you, and they'll know how to go about doing so. If you communicate your needs, your loved ones are more likely to try to meet you halfway. If they want to listen to music, they'll grab headphones. If they were planning to cook up something that will fill the house with strong kitchen smells, they'll pick something else for dinner instead. If there had been plans discussed for later that day, it'll be understood you're probably not going to be participating in the activity. Letting them know how you're feeling lets them know exactly how to be considerate.

This sort of visual system may seem like a wonderful idea, but I want to point out a potential pitfall. When you're going through treatment, you have to be careful not to abuse the mood indicator. It makes senses that you may not be happy often during cancer treatment, but some days will definitely be better than others. For that reason, it's not okay to have that frown up all the time, telling your family and telling yourself that every day is bad. That could easily become a crutch that keeps you from moving forward. It's critical to limit conveying negativity, just like you would limit any negative emotional state. I'm not saying there won't be times when you may need to play the "I have cancer" card. But that will always be my advice on how to *get out* of a bad situation, not how to *stay in* one.

Instead, think of the mood-indicator board as one more way that you *try* to make each day a good day. Some days are going to get away from you, and that happens more often when you don't feel great. Don't beat yourself up about it when it happens. Just commit to trying to make tomorrow a good day. That's the point of focusing on yourself. It's the reason that nobody should expect anything from you. It's also the reason behind making sure you communicate your needs to the people helping you through this. This entire book is dedicated to each of your days being the best day you can have, even if today is a rough one.

Giving the people closest to you an understanding of where you are right now and what you're going through is the most important thing for maintaining your close relationships. I regularly tell myself: "When you're having a bad day, get through it with an eye for the good day that's ahead. Whatever you're feeling, accept that you're feeling it, but really work on limiting the damage it does." I think that goes a long way toward keeping relationships healthy too. Especially with Corinna's and Lorenzo's cancers, we worked as a family on keeping them interested in things beyond their daily pain and struggle. That effort affected all our spirits in a positive way.

* * *

A lot of the people around you will probably understand pretty well when you're experiencing a hard time. They won't expect a lot out of you while you're in treatment. However, some adults and most children simply won't get it. They'll wonder why you can't take out the trash or make them dinner like you always used to do. Over time, even a very reasonable person may begin thinking, *You've been in treatment for months now. Isn't it time you started pitching in around here again?* Left unaddressed, these issues can lead to resentment. Now if you're capable of more activity and movement, then of course you should get up and move. And if you're not there yet, go ahead and see yourself as a person who can turn the corner in the direction of your recovery. But most important, be open about why you aren't doing things like you used to. Let those close to you know if you're honestly scared to go down the stairs with the trash because you're afraid you'll fall. Explain to them that your equilibrium isn't that solid right now. Your blood is thin too, so if you did start bleeding, you'd lose a lot before you could get it under control. Help your loved ones understand that you're focusing on taking care of yourself not out of laziness, but out of self-defense.

Explain to your inner circle that you need so much help from them because the more you do for others, the more your health will suffer. If you have children, this can be an especially difficult thing to get them to understand. Worse, you can't simply tell them to suddenly be self-sufficient if they've never had to be. Maybe they've always had you there to make them a sandwich. Communicate to them that now you need them to make sandwiches for themselves. If you have young children in your care, know this: somebody is going to have to teach those kids how to do the little things for which they've always depended on you. Sometimes it can be you, if you're having a good day. Teaching your kids to make a sandwich shouldn't take too much out of you, and it can be a fun activity that you do together. But remember, too, that it won't *always* be you who does the teaching. People on your support team are going to have to help your kids to learn whatever things it's fair to expect them to handle at their ages.

Children may need to receive some tough love on this point; they can't expect a parent in treatment to coddle them. They have to step up. Kids can do dishes, care for pets, maybe even keep up with the laundry. My own kids loved the feeling of independence they got from learning to do more for themselves. Granted, that wasn't their initial response! Plain and simple, both Lorenzo and Dominic really didn't embrace the prospect of work. Both of them would end up doing more work just to avoid the work they were asked to do, which has always seemed to me so counterproductive. However, Lorenzo and Dominic both really enjoyed some of the meals we cooked at home and wanted to duplicate the dishes during my treatment and then again during Corinna's treatment. This opened an opportunity for the boys to explore cooking, and they did very well! Each mastered his own favorite dish and rarely missed family meals. They came to understand some of the special dietary constraints that came along with treatment, and they even got a little excited learning about how nutrition affected our bodies. Here we are years later, and both men can cook better than every girlfriend they've ever had. I love sharing this fact about them, because to me, it shows how well they turned a potential negative into a total positive. A lot of that depended on how Corinna and I framed those activities. The more we made tasks seem like fun and independent exercises, the more easily the boys took them on. I know firsthand that there are so many opportunities for positive experiences during your cancer treatment. A lot can be good, and even life changing, if you develop your awareness of those little opportunities and welcome them.

You'll be proud of your kids, and they'll be proud of themselves as they master simple tasks. Whatever your children can do for themselves (and maybe for you) will leave less work for the adults around you, and that can help keep your core support team from being overwhelmed by any increase in your needs. The children pitching in will help the adults you count on the most to have more time and energy. That will enable those adults to do things the children simply can't or shouldn't do, as well as take care of the kids themselves.

It may surprise you to learn that your inner circle may not be the only resource you have for helping keep your children happy and out of trouble. During my first week of chemo, I saw an advertisement on a community billboard for Camp Kesem. I can't tell you what an amazing resource that camp was for us. Essentially, college student volunteers provide a one-week summer camp at no cost to you. Everything is paid for with donations. They accepted Dominic and Lorenzo and got them out of the house and away from our dynamic at a crucial moment in my treatment process. At camp, the boys spent time with kids who were also coping with parents who had cancer, and they got to talk and share their feelings about that. Some of their campmates had lost parents to cancer, and everybody learned about that as well as the community resources available to them. It was a great experience for the boys, and it was a relief for my wife and me to have them cared for out of the house while we tried to cope with everything. Usually the camp is a one-time event for younger children; however, our circumstance—years of treatment—meant that Camp Kesem was a summer staple for our kids for several years. It made a permanent imprint on our lives. Lorenzo even became a camp counselor, and when he was undergoing treatment, the Kesem group provided additional support. It's funny how life sometimes goes full circle: one year, Lorenzo was helping younger kids deal with cancer in their families, and the very next year, that same group was there to bolster him.

I want to add that you should also look for resources that are available for your particular type of cancer. Every community has support structures in place that most people don't ever consider. Most of us have heard of the Lymphoma and Leukemia Society and the Susan G. Komen Foundation for breast cancer, but there are a lot of other programs out there to help people with various needs. And there are useful services that have nothing to do with cancer at all. For example, Meals on Wheels isn't specific to any type of disability; rather, it's available to all people in need of a hot meal.

Your community has resources and people who are ready and waiting to help you. It's what they do. And they don't discriminate. They aren't going to ask for your tax return to see if you are down and out enough to deserve their help. They exist solely for your well-being. In fact, there are even services that will prepare your tax return for free if it's that time of year. You owe it to yourself and your family to take advantage of the services that your community has set up to help you through hard times. When you have cancer, you really do need all the help you can get, and you also really need to be proactive about asking for it. Doing so will decrease the burden on your core group and better your odds for a positive result.

Taking charge of your communication with people around you can help to ensure that people know what you want them to know about your condition, that the people who care about you know how best to support you, and that you get the help you need to survive.

CHAPTER 6

ESTABLISHING A TRUSTING RELATIONSHIP WITH YOUR DOCTORS

The bomb just dropped, and you have no idea what the hell is going on. Your cancer diagnosis might be the start of a new experience for you, the experience of feeling like a passenger rather than a driver. If you don't like riding shotgun, this is going to be a tough journey. The plain truth is that your immune system is broken and needs to be repaired. Getting the news that you have cancer is a big emotional hit. I've spoken to cancer doctors who were diagnosed with cancer, and even *they* had the wind knocked out of them.

Imagine if you had known beforehand. You might have done some research and educated yourself about cancer in general and the specific type you're now dealing with. Maybe you would have relocated to a major city with a top-notch medical center or looked more closely at your insurance policy and upgraded your coverage. You also might have started taking your health more seriously than before. I'm sorry to say that nobody gets to do that, at least in the world as it is now. We can envision a future where a single device scans our bodies and detects and fixes anything. Maybe treatments will eventually eliminate all discomfort and pain, have a clear and positive result, and allow us to pick up and go on with our lives without much hassle at all. But that is not how it goes now, and now is when you need to fight for your life.

Your cancer diagnosis might be the start of a new experience for you, the experience of feeling like a passenger rather than a driver.

In all likelihood, your primary care doctor referred you to an oncologist who is a colleague or part of the same medical network. Or your insurance company may have taken charge and assigned you a doctor from its preferred provider list. If you found yourself in the emergency department of a hospital, like I did, the oncologist on call would be your first care provider. My point is that there's a large element of chance determining whom you initially find yourself allied with in your fight against cancer. That part is largely out of your hands, and that is precisely why I recommend that you embrace a practice of trusting those who are assigned to your care.

During my experience and Corinna's, we both questioned whether the doctors assigned to us were our best choice. I think it's natural to resist releasing control to a physician with whom you have no relationship—especially when it comes to responsibility for your life's outcomes. It might be that this step in your life plan demands a quick resolution on your part to honor the partnership with your doctor. Maybe you'll even take a picture of this person who dedicated their life and devoted years of study and experience to helping give you more time on earth. I suggest this, because I feel that I was truly uninformed and lacked any real trust in the medical community. I wish that I had shown some gratitude to the dedicated team giving me a fighting chance to change my life.

Where you were when you got the news wasn't something you could control. Nor is the availability of the best doctors and treatment facilities in your area. Not many of us can pick up our lives and move next door to the best cancer clinics in the world. We have to take what we can get, hope our insurance will cover what we need, or even figure out how to utilize the government health care system to its maximum benefit.

Certain questions will inevitably arise: Is the medical team I'm working with the right one for me? Should I be getting a second opinion? Can I do better than the team I was given? These are all valid concerns. In response to them, I want you to try hard not to let your emotional state cloud your judgment so that you can enter into the relationship with your doctors on your own terms and follow a plan that makes sense for you. How do you make that happen when it comes to the team of doctors assigned to your care? Your treatment plan, for all the ways it seems predetermined, is something of a gray area. It's right at the border of things you can shape and things that are out of your hands.

Your team of doctors will prescribe the best course of treatment possible to give you the best result they are able. Unfortunately, you may not always move forward with that initial plan. Your insurance provider, which is footing the bill, has to get on board. Effectively, your doctors are asking your insurance company's permission to do what they think is best. If you don't have a handle on what your insurance covers and what it doesn't, you're about to receive an education on it. Like their patients, doctors don't have full control over their role in this process either. If your insurance doesn't cover everything, the team works up the next-best plan and presents you with options. If you can pay for some things out of pocket, you get some control back. If you're covering the entire cost of treatments, you have a lot more say in how your team proceeds, but that isn't often the case. For most of us, the procedures we get will be determined by what our insurance will cover.

Even if you had millions to throw at addressing your cancer, this wouldn't bring it fully under your thumb. Money might open up a wider range of treatment options to you, but it doesn't guarantee you a successful result. Many people have the best doctors in the city working with them, and it doesn't affect their chances of survival. The only thing that will get you over this mountain and down the other side is soldiering through whatever sound treatment plan has been drawn up for you.

One thing I highly recommend, even if you have to pay for it yourself, is a PET scan. This type of imaging test creates a detailed map of your body and can detect a wide variety of cancer cells. It also tells your doctors how your organs are functioning, in case they've been compromised by the malignancy. That information can go a long way toward saving your life. I urge you to demand the test and to get it as soon as possible. You want your doctors to have the best information about your cancer that they can get, right from the start. That way, the prescribed plan treats what is actually happening in your body, instead of what they *suspect* is happening. It took me three months to get a PET scan, and that was a lot of wasted time.

* * *

My biggest mistake when I had lymphoma was not trusting my medical team. On the one hand, I didn't want to hear what they were telling me. I thought I could just recharge with blood transfusions and power through my days. I thought I knew better, but I really didn't. I want you to avoid making that same mistake. It's a roll of the dice where you are in your life and what medical team you find yourself with when you get your diagnosis. I urge you to establish trust with them. If you can't do that, then it may be time to get a second opinion and explore other options for care providers. But I wouldn't rush to do that, and I'll explain why.

It's a very subjective thing to decide whether someone is the right doctor for you. You may need a doctor with an amazing bedside manner. Or maybe that personal touch is less important to you than someone's skill and knowledge. Often, people choose a practitioner the same way they choose a presidential candidate: Which one would I rather have a beer with? The important thing is to have a person you can *invest* your trust in. You're going to have to give that trust to them on credit.

One common question that we raise with our doctors is this: "What are my odds at beating my cancer?" Bear in mind that your doctors won't really know *your* odds. When I received my own tentative diagnosis, we couldn't do a Google search for "Ross Suozzi cancer survival rate." Today, I can tell you that it's 100 percent, but when I was diagnosed, that data didn't exist. Your personal survival rate doesn't exist either. No one can know the true odds for your survival, because no one exactly like you has ever gone through precisely what you are experiencing. Those numbers you're hearing may seem frightening, but those odds can still be influenced by what you make of them. Your body is unique, and so are your circumstances. I promise you that whatever odds your doctors present, you probably won't be happy. If they predict a one in ten chance you won't make it, that 10 percent fail rate will seem too high. You'll want absolute certainty, because this is your life on the line. If you're like me, you'll want a prediction of 100 percent success and a do-over if it doesn't work! Of course, your doctors can't give you that, for reasons that aren't their fault.

So where do those odds they quote you come from? Your team will be looking at the collected data from a lot of other people who have had a similar cancer and followed similar treatment to what they're proposing. They'll quote you the percentage chance you will survive based on that, and they will also factor in an assessment of your current health. If the chances for your survival don't sound encouraging, it may be tempting to tell yourself that it's your doctor's problem. You might think that better doctors would quote you better odds. In all likelihood, that wouldn't happen. Those hypothetical "better doctors" would be using the same data from the same sources along with an assessment of the overall state of your health. My advice is to own up to your part in how optimistic your doctor is about your success. Instead of giving in to the temptation to place the blame elsewhere, take responsibility for where you're at now, and consider ways that you can help make your treatment plan work.

Instead of giving in to the temptation to place the blame elsewhere, take responsibility for where you're at now, and consider ways that you can help make your treatment plan work.

Your personal plan for a good outcome has this primary aim:

feed your chances for success, not your odds of failure. From this point forward, make positive choices and cultivate better habits. That's how you can improve your actual chances for success and help determine what your true odds are going to be. Your doctor is there to help you make improvements, and in a best-case scenario, you and your doctor will be working in tandem on behalf of your well-being. You need a trusting relationship with that person or that team of people in order to give yourself your best chances for a successful outcome.

* * *

When cancer shows up, there's a lot to learn and not a lot of time for learning it. As I tried to understand more about my own cancer, it was easy for me to become confused by the dizzying amount of information available and all the new terminology. The two hundred or so known types of cancer are broken down into five major categories: carcinoma, leukemia, sarcoma, lymphatic system cancer, and brain/spinal cancer. From these broad classes, there are branches upon branches splitting off into subclasses and beyond. It's no wonder our heads start to spin when we try to research on our own. Besides that, most of the things you'll find about cancer are not going to make you more comfortable when you read them either. They're going to scare the hell out of you.

Worse than feeling frightened or confused is leaning on bad sources of advice. We live in the Information Age, but not all of that information is valuable or helpful. We all have that uncle or coworker who loves to give "expert" advice, despite not knowing what he's talking about. When I was growing up, I had an Aunt Ruth who would look to TV talk shows and friends for "diagnoses" of her newest pains or health problems. Across the entire world, everyone's know-it-all uncle is on internet message boards giving free advice or promising some sort of miraculous cure. Beware of your susceptibility to that. And even if you are already able to distinguish better from worse sources of information on the web, you should still consider not spending too much time looking up and reading about your symptoms. It is easy enough to access all kinds of information, and you may even find that some but not all of the details mentioned in an online article resemble your personal condition. Indulging your need to know by giving yourself an unguided and speedy online education could perhaps induce additional trauma and anxiety for you. Instead of self-diagnosing your medical condition and how it should be treated, please back away. Give that trust to your medical professionals instead.

If you must occasionally indulge your need to research, by no means should you trust a random person on a message board or put faith in a website for a diagnosis. There are official societies and research databases for whatever type of cancer you're diagnosed with, and these can be good sources of information. If you have access to them, you can use them to educate yourself, or you can simply ask your doctors to gather some of that information for you. I'm advocating for you to trust in your doctors and what they are telling you; although it's good to learn what you can about your condition, you aren't going to become an expert overnight. Your doctors, on the other hand, *are* experts already. They have years of experience and training, as well as access to continuing education on the latest research findings and treatments. Get your answers from them, because they really are your best resource when it comes to medical opinions.

Trust them, too, when they need to collect information from you. Doctors order a variety of tests in order to have hard data and not just a patient's subjective experience to work with. Having a clearer understanding of your schedule for these tests will make the process far easier for you. Use the calendar on your phone to create the outline of events in order to eliminate unplanned surprises. Organize your time to increase what mental capacity you have. I cannot count how many appointments I showed up for at the wrong day or time or even at the wrong location. Your mind will not be as clear as it was before treatment, so make a new habit of keeping a journal or other source of daily reminders to help you eliminate common but costly mistakes like missing a test date or a checkup.

Maybe you aren't being treated at one of the world's leading cancer clinics. That doesn't mean you aren't getting good care from professionals who know what they are doing. Something to bear in mind is that wherever you are, your lead oncologist isn't working alone. I'm not simply referring to the pain management doctor, nurses, and other professionals on the team. I'm talking about the fact that your doctor is able to consult other doctors across the nation and even the globe. You may be receiving treatment in rural Alabama, but your doctor has access to the latest findings from UCLA, the Mayo Clinic, and every other top cancer research center in the world. This is one of the best things about scientists: they share what they know. And they share what has worked in the past. What's more, your doctor is part of a group that might meet several times a week to determine how your treatment is working for you. You never see these people, but videoconferencing and other technology leaves no physician sitting alone, scratching her or his head. Doctors confer with other specialists who all weigh in, offering advice and experience. So in truth, your doctor is part of an entire network of people who have made it their lives' work to treat and cure cancer.

I was treated by Dr. Roberts, a good scientist and someone who knew what he was doing. It was exhausting and overwhelming to arrive at my diagnosis, and it wasn't until my body and my vibrant lifestyle started to deteriorate that we were able to reach a firm diagnosis. My case was extremely different from either Corinna's or Lorenzo's; my diagnosis took months, whereas each of them were provided definitive diagnosis and treatment direction within days. Although Dr. Roberts didn't know exactly how to handle my particular case, he knew whom to contact. People from four different institutions were looking at my blood, working together collectively to draw a conclusive diagnosis for me. I saw Dr. Roberts, but behind the scenes, doctors at the University of New Mexico, several Mayo Clinics, and the Cleveland Clinic shared professional experiences to determine similarities between my case and known non-Hodgkin lymphoma cases. Would I have been right to fire Dr. Roberts because he didn't know immediately what my issue was? No. I would have been making a big mistake that could have delayed getting a proper diagnosis by months.

* * *

It took Corinna and me some time to get comfortable communicating with our doctors about our treatments, and we learned the hard way about *when* we needed to ask questions and precisely *what* we needed to ask. There are going to be some points in treatment when clear communication is really important. I've just talked about diagnosis being one of those moments, as is any time treatment decisions have to be made or new treatment processes are getting underway. Letting your doctors know how much information you need is an important part of establishing and maintaining good communication. And if you have questions but can be shy about asking, write them down, or bring along the person who takes care of you to ask them on your behalf and take notes about the answers. It can be hard to take in all the new information and details when you're just on your own at an appointment; bringing someone you trust with you can go a long way toward getting you the information you need so that you can digest it after your office visit.

When it comes to communicating with your doctors, take the lead. Think about it like this: you simply can't know ahead of time the precise issues your treatment will cause for your body. The same is true of the drugs involved in getting you through the day during your treatment. Every therapy and medication come with a list of possible side effects, but nobody can predict how your body will react, because there are too many variables. One person takes Vicodin and gets good pain relief. The next person can't even keep the pill down and just vomits it right back up. Some people get good results with a drug, and others feel no effects at all. Treatment is a little bit like a game of hurry and wait. The transfer of information is still not instantaneous; during my own treatment, I could sometimes wait weeks for a test result only to find out the results had been sitting on someone's desk for days. Occurrences like this are exactly the ones where the practice of taking control of your life through your Life Plan will be beneficial. Make it a practice to follow up with your medical team. An old-fashioned phone call still goes a long way, especially when your own emotional stability is at risk.

Good communication with your doctors can be helped along by paying attention to your body and learning how to give a clear report about your symptoms. You'll want to be aware of any new health issue that arises and report new discomforts and symptoms to your team. Many times, your doctor will tell you that your symptoms are normal for a majority of patients and not to worry. In the case of something abnormal, letting your team know gives them a leg up on treating it. Early discovery of a new condition can lead to rapid treatment and a better outcome.

I have experienced the unfortunate side effect of a prolonged wait time: a wandering mind. What I needed to do was to focus my personal plan around the facts and information presented by my medical team. Bringing my best-guess self-diagnosis to an appointment was not the way to establish trust with my team. But sharing my symptoms was an effective way for me to work with my doctor to evaluate my treatment plan. Awareness of what is happening in your body during treatment is a powerful tool. Pay close attention to what your body is going through, and try to find words for how it is affecting you. Think about the words doctors sometimes use when they ask us to describe our pain: Is it stabbing? Throbbing? Dull? Does it radiate? Then be proactive about finding the right words or gestures for sharing that information about your experience with your doctors. This kind of reporting isn't complaining; it's the work that's necessary to help your doctors monitor how things are going. You're the only one who can report on how you feel. You may need the treatment to save your life, but you don't need additional scars that might have been prevented by paying attention to your body and giving voice to your concerns.

I believe that if you work on trusting your doctor and your medical team, it will change your overall experience for the better. However, I know there are rare but real situations in which granting or sustaining trust may not be in your best interest, and I know that at the start of any treatment, second opinions can be vitally important for feeling comfortable with all the options before moving forward. If you've really tried but truly can't establish trust with your doctor, or if your personalities are truly mismatched, then it's probably time to make the adjustments to your team. Finding another option will be easier or harder depending on where you live. Then there is the question of whether your insurance will cover treatment with the new doctors you've chosen, especially if they are outside your network. That in itself could be a limiting factor, but if you need a new doctor, you'll have to persevere and find a better fit. You need a lot of trust to get through this difficult and inconvenient time in your life; some of it you have to give on credit, but some of it your doctors do need to earn. Time is of the essence when it comes to implementing a treatment plan, so bear in mind the things I've said, and make a big choice like this quickly if you can.

Come at it with your clearest head and calmest heart. Whatever your decision is, own it and make it work.

As a final word of caution, I urge you to consider your emotional state before seeking another doctor. Finding out that you have cancer, or that your loved one does, is terrifying. Extreme emotions can alter our perceptions and cause lapses in judgment. This is why we try not to drive angry and why we have to take a break from conversations that are getting us too upset. If you've given your doctor a chance and now you're thinking about finding someone else, sleep on it. Come at it with your clearest head and calmest heart. Whatever your decision is, own it and make it work.

CHAPTER 7
MANAGING YOUR PAIN

W e've all had a cold, and likely many of us have had at least one really bad cold or flu. You're clutching your box of tissues, your nose is red, raw at the tip and around the edges; it never stops dripping, and it hurts to wipe. You haven't eaten a real meal in a couple of days, and you didn't taste what you tried to eat earlier today. Eating is work, and having to keep breathing while you're eating requires a lot of effort. Maybe you've got a fever on and off, your body aches, and your gut is sore from clenching your abdominal muscles every time you cough. Your head is pounding, and as your neighbor blasts heavy metal music on loop, you start to wonder if he's trying to drive you mad.

Take whatever experience you have that's like that and stretch it out for weeks and months rather than a couple of days. Maybe it subsides for a day or three, but after each session of chemo, it's back for another four or five. When we have a cold or the flu, most of us aren't too shy about inducing sleep via NyQuil or some other over-the-counter medicine. Honestly, it's no wonder that we turn to opioids so quickly during cancer treatment. We can handle any discomfort or illness if it's over and done soon enough, but when it lingers, or gets worse instead of better, forget it. It's more than tempting to start fishing around in the medicine cabinet for anything that might help. Like a kid exploring his parents' stash of liquor, you can end up digging around for something magical.

As a patient in cancer treatment, the pharmacy doors are flung wide open to you. People doing street drugs will be jealous of you now because you have an all-access pass to the strongest, medical-grade drugs on earth. Your pain management doctor can and will supply you with everything you need, 100 percent legally. Let me explain how this works. Healthcare professionals use a universal pain assessment scale, from zero to ten. Zero is no pain, and ten is the worst pain possible. You tell the doctor where your pain falls at a given moment, from "It's barely noticeable" to "Make it stop!" and in turn, you get the appropriate meds to deal with it. It's as simple as that.

My experience during treatment turned me into a legal junkie. The access I had to hardcore drugs was unbelievable, and my pain during most of the treatment was off the charts.

That's my concern.

* * *

My experience during treatment turned me into a legal junkie. The access I had to hardcore drugs was unbelievable, and my pain during most of the treatment was off the charts. The daily pain radiated from the core of my body to everywhere else. Even my damned fingertips hurt. There was pain from not moving, from wearing clothes, from temperature changes, from walking. Even taking a crap hurt and burned most of the time, as my body was trying to excrete all the toxins I was given to kill the cancer. It's also the case that the disease and the treatment included a wide variety of chemicals and pollutants that, under other circumstances, would have the Environmental Protection Agency setting up a chain-link fence and shuttering a business for hazardous waste pollution. During my treatment, our house was essentially contaminated, and necessary precautions needed to be implemented. As a patient you might not think much about the rainbow-spectrum of fluids you receive, but from administration to cleanup afterward, there can be serious implications for caregivers from secondhand chemotherapy. My only sense of balance throughout all of this came from finding a remedy that would make my body have some moments of peace.

To me, all of the pain felt like it was part of an experiment; each doctor—infectious disease, cardiology, oncology, pulmonary, urology—I think they all were waiting to see when I would pop. On the one hand, the number of pain meds I took each day was relatively consistent. I was usually up most of the night, with Vicodin for quick relief and Percocet for longer-term relief, and I was stacking morphine and two or three patches of fentanyl. This recipe for becoming a real junkie was all legal and all prescribed by my medical professionals. On the other hand, it's also, as you can imagine, a recipe for disaster. This is one of the darkest aspects of treatment, where people with tendencies toward addiction—either because of their personalities or their genetics—risk digging into a deep pit that perhaps they will never dig their way out of.

Reflecting back on it now, I'd say that during treatment,

I experienced three different levels of pain. That first level was a pain that no over-the-counter medicine (at least those available in the United States) could touch. For me, that's the equivalent to something like a deep cut or a severely swollen, twisted ankle. The second level was the equivalent of a broken hip or a piece of metal like a bullet stuck in my arm. Level 3 was where I never wanted to be—a dark and scary place where my body would take control of my mind, and the pain was so constant that no pain management could help alleviate it. I lived with level 3 pain for months, and the level-3 pain meds that I took changed my body permanently. The most significant change was internal—organ deterioration, joint and ligament damage, and the mental imbalance that continues to plague me to this day. If I were giving advice to my earlier self, I'd say, "This is an experience that you need to avoid at all costs." Years later, I still have difficulty accepting the risk-to-reward ratio of that time.

Pain management options—which can include the use of injections, oral drugs, gels, liquids, patches, and whatever else you can think of to reduce or eliminate those horrible feelings—were, and still are, limited, and there is no real safety barrier built into the medication. Unfortunately, at the time of use, it's hard to care what the longer-term effects might be. From my experience, pain relief was absolutely necessary; I had no concern for the future, only the immediate benefit the drug provided. Besides that need for relief, not one professional at any point cautioned me about short- or longer-term effects, especially not the long-term imprint that the pain medicines would make on my body. No one discussed with me the possibility that my future would be permanently different as a result of the long-term, excessive use of pain medication. That's partly, and ironically, because very few studies have been conducted to examine those effects.

* * *

Pain management doctors are relying on you to be honest. They assume it. They can't fact-check what you say. There's no objective way to know if you are at a three but reporting a nine. This is especially true because everyone's pain tolerance is different. Doctors have to trust your description of your pain because if they fail to manage it, that could make your situation much worse. Do they worry about giving you too much? Some of them do, yes. But they have only your word to go by. The system is set up so that you can have access to everything you need. The problem is how often patients may be tempted to indicate that the discomfort is worse than it is. And maybe, at any given moment, that's the truth: "this pain right now" can feel like it's the maximum discomfort you've ever experienced.

Now, if a smorgasbord of legal drugs is not your idea of fun, that's great. If that sounds tempting, all I can do is warn you that you're about to enter a dangerous time in your life. With the phrase "opioid addiction epidemic" plastered across the headlines every day, the reason should be self-evident. But there's still another reason, and it has to do with the trajectory of your illness. You may need even more pain medicine later on just to keep you from losing your mind completely, and the more used to medicine your body is, the more medicine it needs to feel relief. You can actually do yourself a serious disservice in the longer term if you overindulge in the short term.

That's why it's absolutely crucial during this time to be honest with yourself. Ask yourself every day: How bad is my pain, really? Will an over-the-counter pain med take enough of the edge off, or do I need something a little stronger? If you're at an eight or above, I encourage you not to be shy about getting something to bring your discomfort back to manageable. If your body is busy combatting terrible pain, it's going to wear you down and lead to a less positive outcome from treatment. Your doctors want you to get enough drugs to manage the pain.

It's truly a delicate balance between cheating yourself of relief from discomfort on the one hand, and avoiding going overboard and spending every day in a haze on the other. Too much medication, don't forget, can keep you from healing as quickly as you ought to and jeopardize your overall result. Beyond that, if you're drugged out of your mind all the time, your loved ones are going to miss you. Despite you still being in the room, they'll feel like you're not even there. Most important, you won't be getting anything out of life. I've talked a lot about how I hope you will be trying to enjoy yourself as much as you can during the treatment process, and being a zombie isn't going to help that happen. I know that from experience.

During a period of intense pain, I made what some might call an unorthodox decision to conduct an experiment with Lorenzo and Dominic as witnesses. I wanted them to see firsthand the frightening effects of all the pain medications I had been given. "Here's your sad-ass father on the floor fighting cancer. Now let's see what drugs do. Go get me the bottle of pills with the *P* on it. Now watch me take a Percocet and see what happens." Lorenzo and Dominic took note of my dizziness and some shifts in my personality. After an appropriate amount of time, we'd try another drug: "Go get your father a Vicodin," and then later, "Go get the morphine pump." With the latter, they watched me try to count backward from ten and be completely messed up and out of it before hitting six. The kids were surprised by the effects, and surprised, too, at the side effects that made me into a different person or even a barely conscious one. My approach was probably not the parenting most rational people would consider, but my firsthand experience demonstrated to my sons what really happened to me on drugs. I felt the raw demonstration should not be overlooked by my two young boys; I wanted to show them that there was nothing "cool" about my experience, and I hoped that perhaps in the future having witnessed my experience would influence for the better their own personal decision about using drugs.

Another concern with pain medications is the potential for ugly side effects. Personally, I don't think side effects are discussed enough when drugs are prescribed. When I get treatment now at the VA, I typically receive a sheet listing potential reactions to a drug—but it's separate, not on the bottle. The only thing the bottle warns is "Don't take this with milk," or something along those lines. When you're desperate for pain to stop, you're probably not even going to read about a drug's adverse effects. You just sign the form that asks if you've read and understood the information, and then you hope for the best.

It's mind-boggling what sorts of unfortunate side effects can occur. For example, I had an allergic reaction to both oxycodone and hydrocodone. Eventually, I found out that whenever there was opium in my pain management drugs, I'd break out into a severe rash. Of the three different chemical classifications of opioids, there is no option available for me that does not induce an allergic reaction. That meant that in order to benefit from any opioid medication, I had to use injectable Benadryl to combat my allergy. In addition to having to suffer through the allergy and add the Benadryl to my routine, I'd also retain a few pounds of water, so I had to take diuretics to reduce the bloating. Otherwise, for days at a time, I'd look and feel like a corpse someone dragged from the lake. All of that was the result of me taking a pill prescribed for pain. I could get away with one oxycodone, but taking two was risky, and taking it for steady management of pain over a twenty-four-hour cycle was completely out of the question. The drugs meant to relive my pain and discomfort were bringing me more pain and discomfort. I needed better options, but I also knew that I couldn't get by without drugs, as my pain levels were constantly too high.

One thing that helped me was activity. Instead of lying in bed for twenty hours a day, I would get up and move around. Every hour, I'd spend fifteen to thirty minutes up and moving. That helped alleviate some pain, partly by distracting me. This allowed me to cut back on the medications that were causing so many problems and reducing my quality of life. That was one alternative I found to avoid being doped up all day, and I recommend you try it. As another consideration, I want to share with you our experiences with the use of medical marijuana. Those experiences were the direct result of asking ourselves why there is only one pain management program supported by our medical system, without any support for alternatives.

* * *

One of the biggest concerns for Lorenzo's pain management was that we didn't know if he would present addictive traits. After I communicated my concern to Dr. Briggs about that possibility, the oncology staff and I had a discussion of alternative pain management. I was motivated by a genuine conviction that this was the correct path for Lorenzo and knew that I needed to present facts to the staff. I would not say that I received a welcome reception, but they did understand my concerns about addiction. Reluctantly, they agreed to put Lorenzo on medical marijuana, or what is prescribed as Marinol. What I haven't told you until now is that I had already gained some familiarity with it. Believe me: I didn't just decide to experiment on my son. Remember that in the earliest days of my own treatment, before I had a proper diagnosis, I was labeled HIV positive. During that time, I met some interesting people. I was looking for a way out from under the opioid problems I was having, and my new friends introduced me to cannabis suckers. Some of these new friends used to live in San Francisco, where they had cannabis clubs. One of them made confections that contained THC, the active ingredient in marijuana. One day, I was handed a sucker with about ten milligrams of THC and CBD in it. I thought pretty much the same thing as when a doctor prescribed me a synthesized opioid: "If it'll help with the pain, I'll try it."

Let me tell you about precisely how cannabis made a difference. You know by now that I have always worked hard to build both a viable business and a sculpted physique. I'm not interested in compromising either so that I can be high. But when I was given that first THC sucker, I could see immediately that this was going to be a big help. I would pop that sucker in my mouth, and very quickly the pain would subside. It wasn't as drastic as the opioids I'd used (and would later believe I needed to use once my diagnosis had been corrected) but the cannabis made my pain manageable, which is the name of the game. And that pain management came without the ugly side effects that narcotics caused.

I can still remember clearly when I was on all those prescriptions, and it wasn't pretty. I don't have an addictive personality, but I can't say I wasn't getting strung out on morphine and fentanyl. I was rigged up with a shoulder harness pump system that gave me a bump of morphine about every fifteen minutes. A couple of micrograms four times an hour, and I had steady pain management all day long. If things got really bad, I could stack the fentanyl on top of the morphine. The fentanyl came in time-release delivery patches that were good for a few days. I'd have two of these patches on at a time. Underneath the patch, my skin became raw from absorbing the drug. My entire back was raw from those patches. That's how much I was using.

In addition to what was prescribed for me on a steady mainte-nance basis, more was there at my fingertips. If all that medication wasn't enough, I could press a little button on my morphine harness and get an extra bump. I was in pain and drugged silly, so I would push the button and push it again, over and over. I didn't realize at the time that it was controlled to save me from overdose. It's a good thing it was, because Corinna took me in for treatment one day and the nurse said, "You were in some pretty severe pain yesterday." She told me that I'd pushed the button for extra morphine seventy-seven times that day. That's how out of it I was.

Contrast that to my experience with cannabis. I was undergoing chemo at that point, so picture me as a big bald guy with a sucker hanging out of his mouth. Instead of shuffling around like a zombie, I was walking around like Kojak. I was aware, present, and actually in a "Who loves ya, baby?" sort of mood. Most people I'd run across wouldn't have a clue that the sucker was my pain management, so it felt private. I just got to be a person, instead of a drugged-up and checked-out patient. And if I was doing okay with my pain, I'd put the sucker back in the wrapper and save it for later. Compare that with the way I was hooked up to and hooked on the morphine harness and patches. Maybe those suckers weren't strictly legal at the time, but if bending the rules a little gave me that much of an improvement in my quality of life during treatment, I was all for it.

* * *

That's how I came to challenge Lorenzo's pain management doctors when he was diagnosed with leukemia. I'd personally experienced a drastic difference in my ability not only to endure, but to participate in and enjoy my life during treatment, and I wanted my son to have the best of my experience. The fact that not everyone would think I was a good parent didn't deter me. I knew what medical marijuana could be worth to a patient in terrible pain. Lorenzo, by the way, is managing a gym now, not in a grave plot or shooting heroin under a highway overpass. If it seems risky to give marijuana to a teen, all I can say is that our risk paid off.

Let me give you another example, yet another story about my family, but one that I haven't talked about until now. Two years after my treatment had ended and before Corinna's had begun, my mother was diagnosed with stage-four ovarian cancer, and there was little that could be done to save her. Picture for a moment your own mother lying in bed with her eyes rolled back in her head. She's incoherent. You aren't sure she knows you're there. That's how it was for my mom, and what I would see when I visited her. She was on so much pain medication that all she could do was lie there and writhe.

Then I gave her a cannabis sucker. If you remember Lorenzo's transformation after Dr. Abbas gave him the symptom-relief cocktail, my mom's experience was a lot like that. With that sucker, my mother was soon up and functioning. She was alert and interacting with us. She had enough pain relief to make things manageable, and we got my mother back for the time that she had left with us. This is because marijuana gives relief for a number of the specific problems that you run into during cancer treatment. And, like I said, it does this without piling on side effects that undermine the relief you're getting.

* * *

Let's pause here to address the stigma that marijuana carries in the United States. I think we're all familiar with the stereotype of the chronic recreational abuser, the "stoner." Maybe we think of him as an unemployed, unwashed dropout with long hair and a cannabis leaf printed on his T-shirt. He talks about marijuana like some people talk about Jesus Christ. The only time he isn't high is when his dealer is running late. I've met those guys, and I don't think that pot is their real issue. If it wasn't marijuana, they'd be abusing something worse. I don't think the construction worker hooked on oxycontin and operating heavy machinery is much of an upright citizen either. I've been exposed to plenty of those guys too. My point here is that people who habitually abuse drugs aren't good examples of a drug's utility *if that drug is used properly*. I think you'll understand by now that I'm advocating *responsible* use of a drug that has worked well for me, my family, and plenty of others.

The fact that marijuana isn't universally legal in the United States is troubling to a lot of people considering pain management options. At the time I'm writing this, thirty-two states and the District of Columbia have legalized medical marijuana. That's more than half the country, including the seat of our federal government. It's interesting to note that federal law prohibits marijuana use, yet people who work in the federal government's hub voted to legalize medical usage for themselves.

Why is marijuana illegal under federal law? It isn't because people are dying from using it; that simply isn't happening. It's not because of the grave risk of addiction marijuana poses. Compared to the opioid addiction epidemic, that threat just isn't there. And it isn't a "gateway drug," contrary to an argument we hear a lot from law enforcement circles. The argument there goes that using marijuana recreationally will in time lead to using other, more dangerous drugs like morphine, hydrocodone, or any of the other drugs that, when prescribed by physicians, are used with the full protection of the law and are covered by health insurance. Marijuana—the drug our government agencies say will lead to use of those dangerous yet legal drugs—is itself federally illegal and unavailable through your insurance. I just can't see the logic.

It's because the argument that marijuana is a "gateway drug" is not well supported, that the shyness about marijuana in public opinion is best explained not by morals but by following the money. It's no secret that pharmaceuticals are big business. Back in 2014, prescription pain medications were reported to run a total cost of $17.8 billion annually in the United States alone.[1] The total economic burden of pain is an estimated $635 billion annually.[2] That much money buys a lot of political influence. And what do big businesses like to do with their influence? They like to get legislation passed to shut out their competition.

I find this fascinating, so bear with me for a minute while I give you a couple more details. Business competition drove outright prohibition of marijuana in the United States in the 1920s. In 1925, the International Opium Convention was enacted, and it served to maximize the profitability of opioids within the narcotics industry. Namely, the convention pushed for more and harsher regulation of cannabis and shoved it to the periphery. That was capitalism in action. From then on, things kept getting worse for people who wanted to use marijuana for legitimate purposes. The situation reached its lowest point with the mandatory sentencing and "three strikes" laws of the 1980s. Beginning in the 80s, the United States had more people incarcerated for possession of marijuana (even the smallest, most insignificant amounts) than for any other crime. That continues to this day: the ACLU has shown that over 85 percent of the 8.2 million marijuana arrests between 2001 and 2010 were for

---

1   Rasu, R. S. et al. "Cost of pain medication to treat adult patients with nonmalignant chronic pain in the United States." *Journal of Managed Care & Specialty Pharmacy*. September 2014. 20(9):921–928.

2   Chronic Pain Research Alliance: http://www.chronicpainresearch.org/site/index

simple possession.[3] That has been allowed to happen *despite the lack of evidence* that people greatly risk addiction or fatality from using the drug.

Until recently, studies on potential hazards and benefits of cannabis for medicinal use have been scarce, largely due to it being scheduled as a controlled substance in the United States and our government's continued "drug war" policies. For example, if our country gives another nation aid money, that country cannot do medical research on a drug we have classified as dangerous; the United States can and will withdraw its aid dollars. Despite governmentally sanctioned resistance, studies showing benefits of medical marijuana are beginning to come to light. In short, they indicate that the dangers are largely hype.

To the contrary of what we've been told to believe, it's important to point out that people using medical marijuana report reduced nausea and improved appetite. One of the hardest parts of keeping your spirits up during treatment is how much you don't feel like eating. You've got no appetite, you're a little queasy, and you just don't taste anything. Cannabis helps with two out of three of these problems! That can keep patients from wasting away and further compromising their health.

* * *

Another key hurdle during treatment is avoiding depression. Depression is as likely to kill you during treatment as the cancer is. That's one of the reasons why I've stressed the importance of what you do with the twenty-three hours a day you spend outside of treatment. Many people use marijuana specifically to treat depression. They find

---

3   American Civil Liberties Union: https://www.aclu.org/gallery/marijuana-arrests-numbers

that it helps them maintain an elevated mood and alleviates anxiety and other symptoms. Consider how that stacks up against pharmaceuticals like Prozac, the side effects of which include weight gain and loss of sex drive. How well is something fighting depression if it's giving the depressed person more to be depressed about?

Medical marijuana provides relief from the pain that keeps cancer patients bedridden, helps them maintain a healthy weight, relieves nausea, and improves mood—all at a time when those things are profoundly necessary for survival. If that sounds appealing, I encourage you to explore it as a serious option. You don't have to smoke anything if you are averse to that. Personally, I need my lungs healthy for other things. Many edible THC varieties are available, from cookies to candies. And remember, this is probably the one time in your life where you don't have to worry about calories. You're going to need them to keep your weight up.

Maybe medical cannabis is for you, and maybe it isn't. That's not for me to say. What I want is for you to decide for yourself, instead of letting an insurance company or a pharmaceutical lobby dictate what your pain management plan should be. Unfortunately, being turned down by insurance is a real concern. Your doctors can come up with the best plan, and the insurance company can say no. Maybe your pain management doctor is open to you trying synthetic THC, but your insurance carrier is not.

A common objection to medical marijuana is that most insurance companies won't pay for it. Let me just say this. If your insurance refuses medical marijuana products, you're going to have to decide if using them for pain management sounds appealing enough for you to pay for them out of pocket. Like I said, I did, and I have no regrets. Everyone's situation is different, just as all of our bodies are different, but I urge you to weigh whatever information you can access and decide for yourself what will give you a better experience.

* * *

I know from experience that it can be hard to talk with your doctor about this issue, especially if there are concerns over the legality of medical marijuana where you live. When Lorenzo was in the hospital for treatment, I saw drug-sniffing dogs go up and down the halls. We never had any problems with Lorenzo or any of his friends getting in trouble with the law, but facing that possibility can be scary. If your instinct is to lie to your medical team about your decision to try medical marijuana, my advice to you is not to do that.

> *Trying to hide from your doctors something you're taking into your body is like a kid hiding something under the mattress. Sure, he thinks his parents don't know, but that's only from his own inexperience.*

Trying to hide from your doctors something you're taking into your body is like a kid hiding something under the mattress. Sure, he thinks his parents don't know, but that's only from his own inexperience. Anytime you provide a urine sample, your doctors are doing tests. Maybe they're running a pain management panel to check the levels of the drugs they've prescribed. They aren't being sneaky; they just want, and *need*, to know if you're taking your meds properly. They may also be running a nine- to twelve-panel drug screen, meaning they're testing for nine to twelve different substances. This tests for all the usual illegal things people abuse as well as a few over-the-counter items they might be concerned about. Why do they do this? Because *they know patients lie to them.* A doctor will ask what you're taking, hoping you'll be forthcoming but knowing full well it's possible you're going to hide something. It doesn't even have to be something illegal! How many people do you think honestly report how many alcoholic drinks they have a week during a physical? So be aware that doctors test for drugs as a matter of routine, and remember that their doing so is a good thing for you overall.

If you're being treated for a condition that's known for being painful, you can be confident that your doctor is running a pain management panel. That tests for the ordinary substances found in a drug panel but will also have something extra. A normal drug test shows how much of something is in your system. Because people metabolize things at different rates, a pain management panel has an element of interpretation. Let me explain. Most medical tests are currently automated. In the case of a pain management panel, an analyst interprets the raw data and tells the doctor what the varying levels of substances mean. That's like trying to hide something from a CSI investigator. If you're lying about using medical marijuana, you're probably not fooling your doctor, and you're definitely not fooling the analyst. To convince you, I'll tell you one reason why they aren't easily tricked. A typical drug screen will also measure levels of creatinine. That's a substance you make in your body during metabolism and excrete in urine. If your urine is extra diluted from drinking a lot of water or adding water to a sample, they'll know. Then they adjust for the levels of creatinine that ought to be in your sample and see how much to scale up the numbers of other substances.

I've heard of doctors writing in the notes on their charts that a patient repeatedly, consistently tests positive for cannabis but continues to lie about it. What does the physician do about it? She shakes her head and keeps an eye out for anything that might cause a health concern. That's her job. She monitors what drugs her patients are actually taking. She keeps tabs on what concentrations are present in samples to keep patients safe from harmful interactions or other complications like overdosing. This is why my advice about telling your doctor you're considering cannabis for pain management is to relax, take a deep breath, and be honest.

I've never heard of a doctor turning someone over to law enforcement. Doctor-patient confidentiality and HIPAA prevent that from happening. No doctor is going to go against that and lose her right to practice medicine. Doctors are there to fix the medical issue you brought them, not influence your whole life.

President Reagan's drug war hindered research on cannabis for a long time, but marijuana has clearly started to gain mainstream acceptance as a valuable tool. Doctors know this. Chances are good they're aware that a number of their patients have made the same choice, whether they disclosed the fact or not. If you open an honest dialogue with your doctor about your decision to try cannabis for pain management, you may be surprised. And whether or not you are interested in cannabis, having an open and honest dialogue with your doctor about the use of opioids for managing your pain is an equally good thing to do.

CHAPTER 8
PROTECTING YOUR LEGACY

U p to this point, we've focused on safeguarding your health and protecting your relationships, all with the intention of helping you survive and even thrive during treatment. Your survival deserves your attention and your full effort. If you've decided to reprioritize your life and take care of yourself, you can't give it less than your best. Now I want to switch over to thinking about how to protect what's yours. In order to safeguard what you've built over the years or whatever you have now, you'll need to reach out to some people who could care less about your condition, like lenders and bankers. You'll likely have to have some hard conversations and make some tough choices. There are going to be things you have to let go of, so that you can hold on to what matters most.

The simple fact of cancer that no one prepares you for is this: your income decreases, and your expenses go up. There is no way to avoid this unfortunate situation. My approach to this issue was my biggest mistake. I was swinging at a piñata fully blindfolded and with no idea how high my target was hanging. I've said that an important part of your life plan for treatment is to be flexible enough to accommodate changes that are likely to crop up. Believe me when I say that your Life Plan must include emphasis on financial flexibility as well. If there is just one thing you take away from this entire book, let that be it. Create as bulletproof a plan as you can to successfully navigate through the financial element of cancer treatment. Plan for the worst, and get advice from a financial planner, accountant, or other factually informed adviser as early as you can.

I'm guessing that you've built something for yourself and those you love that's worth protecting. I'm talking about your legacy. If you are a parent, that should be a familiar concept to you. You want your children to have a better life than you did. You try to give them the advantages that you didn't have growing up. You try to build something that you can pass on to them to give them a leg up on life. For example, maybe you've set up a college fund for them. That's a great legacy. You've probably also moved up in the world from your very first job as a teenager, and you have some things to show for it. Maybe you own your house. Instead of putting rent money in someone else's pocket each month, and being no better off, you're building equity. Every time you pay your mortgage, you're financially better off than you were last month. Maybe you want to have money to care for your spouse, for your aging relatives, and for yourself as you age. That's a personal legacy too. Whatever you've got, I want you to think about how to hold on to it.

I've worked to develop a legacy to pass on to my family. I want the people I love not to have to experience the same difficulties I did. It's an old story and maybe much like yours. My grandfather came to the United States from Palermo, Sicily, at twenty years old with twenty dollars in his pocket. After he arrived, he started selling linens door to door. In time, he bought a car and peddled sheets and towels out of the trunk. After a while, he bought a house—and then a better house—and raised four children. The next generation, including my mom, had the privilege of going to private schools. Some of them went to college and had brand-new cars at twenty. They had a lot fewer worries because those who came before them had worked to build security for them. That hard work, and my parents' contributions to that security gave me the luxury to do things like marry for love and work in a skilled trade. My life was a step or two up from my grandfather's because of what he did and passed on to me.

In turn, my wife and I took some risks and got our own business going. As I write this, I'm splitting my time between our gym and getting Lorenzo set up with a gym of his own. I've put a lot of time and labor into renovating Lorenzo's space so that he can have a good business of his own to manage. This is how we all tend to hope things go from one generation to the next. But it's easy during a time of hardship like cancer treatment to lose the things you've worked for. If you're not smart and quick about doing what needs to be done, the next generation can wind up right back where you started or, if you aren't careful, even worse off.

During my treatment for lymphoma, I went through a lot of hardship because I was trying to protect the business Corinna and I had built. Our bank did not care about us. They didn't care how long and hard we had worked to make our business successful. They had no idea how many hours of our lives we'd invested in our gym, and they wouldn't have been interested if we'd told them. They knew there was profit to be made. All they had to do was take away the business my wife and I had dedicated our lives to creating. If they had managed to do that, they might have slept like babies on their big pile of money. I went through a lot of effort to keep the bank from knowing what was going on in my life. I was stressed and scared every day: they kept harassing me with phone calls, and I kept pretending I wasn't sick. Remember, I took many of those calls in the hospital bathroom, with my rear sticking out of my hospital gown.

I want to help you not to have as hard a time as I did.

I want to help you not to have as hard a time as I did. By avoiding certain pitfalls, you can make holding on to what you've built for yourself and your family a lot simpler.

* * *

The first thing I want to impress upon you is that *you must act quickly*. I know that your mind is occupied. You have a new ache this morning. Your skin smells weird. Food doesn't taste like anything, and you can hardly swallow anyway. Your big toe is so swollen, your shoes don't fit. You're trying to figure out what is going on with your body and keep yourself alive. Nevertheless, what I need you to do now is step outside your present discomforts and think about your future. A little action now will help save the things you've worked so hard for. If you put off doing the things I'm going to recommend, you're likely to have problems. Those problems, once they get started, are going to snowball faster than you would believe. Surviving cancer is a big deal. It's a huge win. Surviving cancer without becoming broke and homeless is even better.

In other words, you may already have worked hard, but now

you're going to have to keep working so as not to lose what you have. You won't be able to perform as usual while you're in treatment, and you'll probably be out of action for a while. Let's be conservative and say you'll be unable to work for about sixty days. That's a very optimistic estimate, and you could easily be away from work for much longer. How is that going to affect your life?

Your overhead doesn't go down if you get sick. You still need to pay your mortgage, make your car payment, keep the lights on, and everything else. And I'm sorry to say this, but even with great insurance that pays for just about everything, there's still a deductible to be met and copays to deal with. When you go in for treatment, you'll have to hand over some money right there and then. So your ability to work and earn has gone down, but your overhead has actually gone up. Some pretty simple arithmetic leads us to the big question: If I have more bills and less money, who doesn't get paid?

Considerations like these are critical, and you'll need a plan for when they arise. I'll share with you how I approached these problems, but your own case is likely to be different, and you'll need to take stock of your own situation. Unfortunately, there's no cookie-cutter solution that I can hand you. Just like developing your plan for your other twenty-three hours, there just isn't a "one size fits all" solution. My hope is that if you're front-loaded with more information, your decisions will have a much better chance of being the right ones for you.

During the early stages of my treatment, our personal and business finances were stressed to the maximum. Our debt load was enormous, my ability to earn was undermined, and the bank was sniffing around our door every day. Unless every moving part in our financial machine worked in sync, the whole thing would go up in smoke. Our gym and our dreams would be stripped from us and sold at auction.

This was 2007, and the country's economic downturn was only just beginning. Despite that, the projections of business growth for our new gym location were good. The data suggested that our debt should be completely supported, and with some modest growth, we would soon become profitable. Nobody predicted the construction shutdown on our complex, though. We didn't foresee the legal fees we'd spend to get the building process restarted either. It wasn't a great way to enter into the early stages of what people refer to as the Great Recession. As we've discussed, that level of stress did nothing to help me with my struggle toward recovery.

In the first few months of my treatment without a proper diagnosis, my physical ability to work was cut down to 10 percent. This meant that I had more time than ever before in my life to sit and plan. My mental capacity for work was cut down to about 50 percent, but I made that be enough. I spent that time and brainpower making a plan to protect everything that was so close to slipping through our fingers.

Corinna and I have always been responsible business owners. Whenever we were short on funds, we'd work harder or work more hours. That was our instinct, and it had carried us through a lot of years. This time, though, Corinna was already doing all she could by picking up the slack for what I was unable to do. Working harder or longer wasn't going to happen, and that left me in unfamiliar territory.

On the worst days, I considered what all the financial professionals advised: I thought about filing for bankruptcy. I know that it's a legitimate business tool and it lets people start over, unburdened by debt. A lot of highly successful people have done it, often multiple times. To me, it seemed immoral. Worse, it felt like embracing failure. How do you calmly accept what you've struggled your entire adult life to avoid? When I imagined myself handing in the bankruptcy papers, I had this vivid image of myself sitting in the electric chair, the lights dimming for a second when the power flipped on. The best advice I could get from professionals was that we were very unlikely to come out of bankruptcy with our gym. It would have been the death of our dream, and I'd be the one throwing the switch. I just couldn't do it.

We couldn't make extra money by working more, and I refused to risk losing the gym in bankruptcy court. What other option did I have? I decided that we needed to be smarter about the money we already had. I examined each of my family's financial responsibilities so I could determine a prioritized list of essential payments. Dave Ramsey or Jim Cramer weren't going to tell me that I needed to do that, but I knew. Maybe it was partly because I was high on prescribed opioids, but I was ready to make some bold choices. I was playing for the survival of my family's dreams. With that on the line, I needed a plan for success. What I came up with was unorthodox enough to make an accountant or financial advisor deeply uncomfortable, and it might not be for you. I recognized that there would be some collateral damage caused by paying some people and not paying others. Neglecting debts would have consequences, and it did. The gym wasn't an acceptable loss, so I had to choose what I was willing to lose to keep it. I made some tough decisions that negatively affected my credit score.

If you've been working your whole adult life to get your credit score up, let me just say this: this is one of those times in your life where your control over outcomes is seriously limited. You can't save everything, so you save what matters most. Your creditworthiness is not what matter most. That might be hard to swallow. Just like I couldn't accept bankruptcy, abandoning your FICO score might seriously challenge your notion of being a responsible adult. If you feel some pride about your score, you're not alone. A good credit score gives you a sense of security and prosperity. But what does that number really mean? A higher number tells you that you can go deeper into debt more easily. That's it. Your credit rating doesn't mean anything to anybody except for the banks.

Let's walk through a scenario. We'll say you have a $10,000 credit balance and a minimum monthly payment of $156. You can't make that payment because you don't have money coming in, or you have reduced income, and there just isn't enough. The next thing you know, you're thirty days late. You still can't make that payment. Forty-five days go by, and they lower your credit rating. If you're like most everybody else, you're going to stress about the score you worked to establish. Most likely, though, you always made your payments on time because you wanted your magical number to go up. Probably, you made your payments because you could afford to. In other words, your credit rating went up solely as a byproduct of making regular payments. The fancy algorithms they use to determine good or bad credit include the percentage of credit you have available versus how much of that you're currently using. The moment you went into the hospital, your credit score took a hit. The moment you put some prescriptions on your card, you took a hit. The more credit you take advantage of to take care of yourself in your time of need, the worse your credit score will get. My advice is this: just let it go.

If you don't, you're going to make mistakes you can't afford. You're going to make that $156 payment. After all, you've got a nest egg, right? So you'll dip into your bank account to protect your credit score. Maybe you've put a little something away each month for years as your rainy-day fund—and it's raining *now*. It may never rain again as hard as it started raining the day you got your diagnosis. Earlier, I recommended that you spend the money that you do have on living as best you can. And I mean that, especially in terms of the decision to engage in the treatment process rather than avoid it. Here, though, I want to qualify my advice. It's time to use your savings as a life raft. Hang on to it as tightly as you can. If you think your nest egg will be all it takes to get you through to the other side of treatment, the chances are high that you're wrong. Everybody's case is different, but I'm willing to bet that your out-of-pocket expenses for treatment alone will be more than you anticipate. Unless your health insurance is absolutely amazing, I estimate that you have a $5,000 deductible. So take five thousand away from your savings right off the bat. What percentage of your nest egg just left the nest? A fifth? Half? If your rainy-day fund is still looking healthy, good for you, but chances are good that it's been cut substantially. That should concern you, because there's still more to subtract.

You know to expect medical bills, and maybe you've planned well for them. But things you don't anticipate will pop up. Your feet swell, so you need new shoes. Your skin is so sensitive that you have to buy new shirts—the softest you can find. These may seem like spur-of-the moment needs, but they are going to make a huge difference in your comfort level and your overall well-being. I suggest that you avoid spending cash for these items too. If you don't put these things on credit cards, your savings will be gone in no time. Think of your nest egg as your last resort. Whatever cash you have saved, do not touch it. This is one of the most important pieces of advice I have to share with you. Hold off on spending even a cent of your savings.

There are tough decisions to make. Can you live without a phone? Most of us don't feel like we can, because we need to stay in touch. Internet access? Maybe you can use free Wi-Fi somewhere. You'll have to figure out what works for you. Identify what you have that you can monetize. Do you have spare transportation, like a motorcycle you aren't riding or that classic car you keep telling yourself you'll fix up someday? Liquidating or selling your personal items during this time can be demoralizing, so plan on resorting to that only just before dipping into your savings. That said, if the television in your bedroom can buy you another week's worth of immune suppressants and antibiotics, sell it!

* * *

While I was going through treatment, our overhead was enormous from trying to keep a business afloat. We borrowed money from everyone we could. Family members, gym members, you name it. Anyplace we could get a loan to keep things running and seeming like nothing was wrong, we did it. And it worked, with a few hiccups. One of those hiccups was particularly mortifying. During that time, we threw our son Dominic a birthday party, and the electric company shut off the lights. They threw the switch and cut us off when we had fifteen or twenty kids and their parents over.

Even given the hiccups we experienced, my message to you is to do what it takes to hold on to your rainy-day fund. Don't spend a dime of it until you truly have no other way to pay for something that's going to keep you alive. When you can't get anything on credit anymore, you're going to need that cash. If you spent it up front, trying to protect your credit score, it's not going to be there when your credit falls apart anyway. Your cash is king, and once it's gone, you're going to be out of options. Leveraging your credit is one option to keep your money in your own pocket as you deal with the mounting costs of treatment. Another way is applying for financial hardship wherever you can. That can help keep you from defaulting on anything from your student loans to your mortgage. Whoever you normally make payments to, find out immediately what you can do to reduce those payments or put them on hold.

This, too, requires active communication on your part. Taking initiative here can be the difference between keeping a firm hand on the wheel or your finances spinning out of control. Your electric company, for example, doesn't know about your condition. Until you explain your situation to them, they don't even know you're ill, much less unable to work. Many power companies have payment deferral programs. A program like this could have eliminated the lights going out during my son's party. The critical thing is to reach out. If your utility companies have any sort of deferral program, get that working for you from the start. Knock on the doors of the companies you do business with, and you may be amazed at the opportunities that open up. Every minute you spend in communication with your mortgage servicer or landlord is enormously valuable, because maintaining stability in your environment, in your household, is essential during treatment. It's not uncommon for a patient in treatment to make payments late or even miss them. This happens even with the best support team.

Remember when the president of special assets at our bank told me that I'd exceeded my "personal capacity"? He had no idea what I was going through. He didn't know where I was during those phone calls or the condition I was in. I hadn't let anyone at the bank know about my illness, and I had even gone to great lengths to hide my condition from them. And then there we were in that phone conversation. I was crushed by the reality of being insolvent and the stress it was causing at such a critical moment. And I contributed to the pain of that moment by being convinced that the bank shouldn't know a thing about what I was going through.

Don't let something like this happen to you, especially when it comes to the place you live. Think about it like this instead: when you entered into a loan agreement, you and your lender became partners. The same goes with any type of lending agreement. You're an asset to your lender. That's good news, and it means that losing your dwelling (mortgaged or rented) is a long way away if you talk with them. To ensure that you continue being an asset, they built certain contingencies into your mortgage or lease. In fact, they set up options for just the kind of situation you're in. What's available is going to vary by institution, so reach out to yours and find out what they have to offer. They don't want you to default, so talk to them and get the best deal you can to save your home.

Prioritizing your home is critical, because whatever you may feel like you can sell off or live without, you still need a place to live. You want to come home to your own bed and a familiar environment. There's nowhere else you can have the level of control over your life as you have in your own home. And if you've ever spent a night in the hospital, you know how much it's possible to appreciate the comforts that being at home offers.

When you're working to maintain your home is exactly when you should draw attention to your cancer. Communicate to your mortgage servicer or landlord exactly what you're going through. Tell them that you need to stay in your home so you'll have the best chance of survival. Be up front about the fact that your finances are going to be strained for a bit. But emphasize that your goal is to be back working as soon as you can. If you're living in an apartment, remind them of how long you've been a good tenant. Most people are people first and employees second, so give the people you talk to a chance to show they have a heart. If that fails, appeal to their business sense. Having you potentially making a late payment is better than an empty apartment bringing in nothing. I strongly recommend that you overcome any shyness you might have about letting these folks see the condition that you're in. Look them in the eyes, call them by their names, and force them think of you a human being, rather than just an apartment number or account number. I also can't recommend strongly enough that you do this well in advance of missing a payment. Build the relationship with them early on in your treatment process in case you need to call on them later. The worst thing you could do is avoid these conversations or put them off until the last possible second. If there's any chance of hanging on to what you have, you need to set your plan in place and act on it. Delay is going to cost you things you can't afford to lose; being proactive is going to help you keep your life intact.

Just like when you customized your plan for living, you'll need a financial plan tailored to your needs and tailored to protect your assets. Having that plan will reduce the stresses on you during treatment and set you up for a better outcome. The steps I took myself won't be right for everyone, but some elements will likely be of value to you. If nothing else, start thinking strategically along these lines and *prioritize* your finances. And just to be clear: by no means am I encouraging you to ignore your financial obligations. That isn't a plan; that's just hiding from reality.

Keep in mind, too, that you're not the only one who is going to be affected if you don't act in a timely way. Whatever else you've built in your life, you've also built relationships with people who depend on you in one way or another. Even if you live a simple life farming your couple of acres, you have attachments. You have a crop and people counting on that crop reaching the market. If you disappeared one day or just can't make good on your commitments, people are going to be affected. What you have also connects you to other people. And on that note, don't forget that there are people-powered organizations and programs (both local and national) that may be able to help you pay for treatment or even just get transported to your treatment if that becomes an issue for you. And in some cases, there may be opportunities to participate in clinical trials and other cutting-edge treatment options that often require no payment from patients.

Many of you likely have more connections than a truly solitary person. As someone who took pains up front to make sure to hold on to what I had, I can tell you that I looked around for anything and anyone that could help. And I don't regret taking that approach. We needed to hang on to the things we had and to make the whole process more manageable and less painful. I want you to do the same. Reach out for whatever lifelines you have available. Take advantage of options anywhere they present themselves to help you get through this with your legacy intact.

CHAPTER 9

LIFE AFTER CANCER

I've shared with you some of the physical and mental aftereffects of my time in treatment that I'm still dealing with, years out of recovery. These problems are largely personal and normally painful for me to talk about. I am pushing through that because I want to use my mistakes and challenges to help warn you, so you can have the mental toughness to weather whatever comes your way. I believe that if you're better prepared for what could happen, you'll have better outcomes and fewer scars than me.

After recovery, I was eager to resume my precancer lifestyle. Often, though, the aftereffects of treatment changed how I could perform tasks. I was reaching for a level of freedom that I hadn't had in a while. I couldn't wait to go hiking and get back on a mountain bike. I could do those things, but the cost was high. I overdid it on my first hike and knocked myself out of action for the rest of the week. When I got on the bike again, I had to moderate how much

I did of that as well. It was then that I learned the importance of budgeting my energy.

* * *

If the things you want to do straight out of recovery are fairly strenuous, don't be disheartened. When you're craving freedom, even a simple trip to the supermarket can give you a taste of that. The normalcy of it can be good for you too. During treatment, the grocery store may have been a place to avoid, but now it's time for a triumphant return to the cereal aisle. I recommend you use trips like this to dip your toe in the water of regular activity and see how your body reacts. How good is your mobility and balance? Are you mentally and emotionally prepared to return to being surrounded by strangers in uncontrolled conditions?

You may need to consider physical or mental challenges that you may not have expected as you resume your previous routines. Count on that and prepare yourself. The sooner you come to terms with your new ability levels and limitations, the better your life will be going forward. Are you struggling with reduced memory function, or as people call it, "chemo brain"? Like a reduction in hand-eye coordination, or lessened physical stamina, this may be something you'll have to adapt to as you work on resuming your familiar life.

We only have so much energy. It was true before cancer, but it becomes especially apparent afterward. I work on being mindful of the physical energy I have on a given day and setting realistic goals for myself. Knowing that I have to budget my energy, and how much I can spend without overexerting, is critical for my ability to make good decisions. I remind myself daily not to worry about how much longer it takes me now to walk up a flight of stairs. I force myself to take one step at a time and to watch my feet placement. The time I could save getting to the top won't mean anything to me if I fall and shred my tender skin. Pretending I'm the same as I used to be isn't worth the pain of my body reminding me that I'm not.

Do what you can now, with the body you have today. Then do the same thing tomorrow and the next day. Like me, you might not be able to do some things you love as often or for as long. But you're going to be around to continue doing them. More than that, you still get to explore life and find new passions. You get to try new desserts, hike new trails, and try out new hobbies that you never made time for before now.

> *Do what you can now, with the body you have today.*

* * *

There are a few other guiding principles that I try to practice daily. I want to share them with you so that you can be unstoppable, whether you are still in treatment or have completed it.

GRATEFULNESS

A daily practice of conscious gratitude can serve you well after treatment. It's harder to get bogged down by what we don't have when we're giving thanks for the second chance that we've won. Remember how fortunate you are, and project that into the world every day. Everyone knows somebody who doesn't realize how good they have it. But if gratitude is part of your persona, you'll be more content and maybe even more charismatic. You owe it to yourself to be that person and also to understand that now there is little preventing you from achieving any result you envision. The wall in front of you that seemed so insurmountable might now appear only knee high. When we aren't afraid to fail, what was once overwhelming becomes manageable.

HUMILITY

The feeling of personal achievement that comes with being a survivor is one I find difficult to describe. That feeling may be difficult for even your inner circle to comprehend. They may see that this experience has changed you, but they can't fully appreciate how. Friends and relations in the outer circles of your social sphere will have even less chance of any meaningful understanding. As a survivor, you need to recognize that most people you encounter will never understand your journey.

Oddly enough, there's a warrior's strength to be drawn from that feeling of being connected to others in our shared vulnerability.

This awareness will help you eliminate a wide variety of scars that would otherwise cloud your new lifestyle. While you can't expect others to comprehend your treatment and recovery journey, you *can* practice being a humble presence, which will evoke a level of respect from everyone your life touches. Too often, our game faces are arrogant ones, as if everyone around us belonged to the opposing team. We posture and curate a public image of strength and competence in which we imagine ourselves as better than other people. But as cancer patients, we are frequently reminded of the fragility that we all share. When you're lying on a gurney, lined up with four other people waiting to get a CT scan, the truth becomes clear: you're the same as the person next to you.

Remember that as you recover. Keep in mind that feeling of being fragile and humbled, surrounded by others feeling the same way. Oddly enough, there's a warrior's strength to be drawn from that feeling of being connected to others in our shared vulnerability.

Your strength can give comfort to others, provided you bear in mind that you're no better than them. The moment you become arrogant and think you are above others, you cut yourself off from those around you. Then, you stand alone in a lie, and this helps no one, you least of all. A humble attitude and awareness that we all have our struggles will bring out the same awareness in others. That can help you foster the sort of supportive environment that will help you feel more and more like you're participating in the life you want for yourself.

ACCEPTANCE

To keep emotional scarring at bay, cultivate acceptance of what's happened in your life. Avoiding the "why me"—the victim syndrome—applies equally much posttreatment as it did at diagnosis. Accept what was out of your hands, but recognize that you're now more capable than ever of taking charge of what you can control today. Not every survivor chooses to embrace this mentality. Often, negativity eats at survivors, and defeatist thinking sends them down a self-perpetuating spiral of angry thinking. We spoke early on about limiting the time we give to negative thinking, feeling anger or resentment, and indulging other destructive emotions. Beyond treatment, this same practice must be maintained. Building on the practice of containing and reducing negative thoughts should continue for the rest of your life. Restrict the time you allow yourself to indulge self-pity, doubt, anger, or any of the rest. Use that time and energy for better things, like appreciating those you love.

I had a striking dream not too long ago that involved dying and the feeling of mystery that surrounds death. During my cancer treatment, I battled so hard against death that I refused to wear a shirt with a skull on it that my wife bought for me. My skin was so sensitive that I could hardly bear to wear clothes, and that extra-soft shirt would have been just what I needed. But I refused to even appear to embrace what I was fighting. I realized when I had that dream that I can now embrace the idea of death. That's a positive achievement for me. After what I've been through, I'm just not afraid of it anymore. I believe that you will come to that same place of acceptance and courage. When you do, you can harness the energy most people invest in being afraid. You can channel it into a positive daily activity, and it will propel you past whatever obstacles you may face. People who haven't been through cancer will never have this tool that you and I share. We can harness that deep-down desire that we once applied to merely staying alive and direct it into tangible personal achievement.

AVOIDING OTHERS' NEGATIVITY

If you are anything like the rest of us, there are negative people in your life. Beware of their negativity, doubt, and anger. Don't give them your precious energy or your irreplaceable time. Negative people are best handled like your own negative thoughts. Like stray animals, if you don't feed them, they will stop coming around so much. That said, even with the positive and loving people in your life, you may have to be careful how much you give of yourself. Your mental and physical resources are limited. One of the ways you survived cancer was by focusing on what you truly want and need. Keep that going. Be a little selfish with your energy when you know that doing so will not harm anyone else. You fought your way to another chance at life.

I'd say you've earned the right to use that chance to keep making decisions that make you happy.

* * *

I want to speak directly to the benefits of various forms of therapy. I didn't mention it before now because I honestly think that its value actually increases after cancer treatment is over. Some people go through treatment with very little physical scarring. In fact, a patient may have more emotional scars after their battle with cancer than they had physical discomfort during the process. Emotional scarring is something we don't see outright, and because of that, it can be challenging to address. For example, any one of us may come away from treatment experiencing a serious identity crisis and wondering who we are now.

On the news, you see guys with prosthetic limbs running marathons or playing sports all the time. You see Lance Armstrong, a hero to a lot of people, my sons included, whose legendary prowess was only enhanced by his battle with advanced testicular cancer. You don't see the depressed person on the news or the PTSD sufferer whose emotional scars have changed his or her life. But it's often the case that those who have been through cancer treatment will seem more reserved afterward, less willing to open up and share themselves. That's because things that happened during the process have done some emotional damage.

Emotional scars from one source or another are common in survivors. You'll remember me saying that during my cancer treatment, it was important to me that I take personal responsibility for many things, including monitoring my own emotional state and behavior. By paying attention to these things, I learned I could adjust and adapt to the new environment I found myself in during treatment. Well, those challenges didn't disappear after treatment ended. The expectations others placed on me and my own attempts to understand and deal with the different personalities I encountered each day continued to be challenging. I needed to keep working on getting back in balance as a man, a husband, and a father. I take each of these roles very seriously, so I enlisted professional help.

There are many therapeutic options, and I've tried nearly all of them. The most common approach is group therapy. Not coincidentally, this is the least expensive form of treatment. Group therapy can be a useful tool for giving survivors a sense of community. Talking with others who are facing very similar challenges can help group members see that others understand what they are dealing with. Also, there can be an element of cohesive purpose, as participants work together toward common goals. The idea with group therapy is to share experiences, give support, and provide positive feedback. It's possible to learn a lot about your own struggles as you help others deal with theirs. Creating a bond with other survivors and forming a team can give each member of the group better resources for their own healing. If the personalities in the group can work together constructively, this can be an excellent option for managing your scars.

In some cases, individual counseling can be combined with group sessions to focus more time on your specific needs. One potential drawback of group therapy, as you might imagine or already know, is the time spent working to aid the other group members. This can be beneficial, but it can just as easily eat away the time and energy you need to work on yourself. Individual talk therapy will be more expensive than group, but 100 percent of the time is focused on your individual improvement. And depending on your personality type, individual talk therapy might be vastly more effective.

If your scars are the kind that can be addressed by changing your thinking surrounding a given issue, you might choose to embrace cognitive behavioral therapy (CBT). This helped me personally, and is nowhere near as scary as it might sound. CBT is a system of restructuring patterns of thought. Learning more about my own behavioral patterns and some of my triggers gave me a better idea of what works for me and what doesn't. Exploring this type of therapy can lead to new learned behaviors that allow you to face your scars and problems head-on, rather than avoid or bury them.

Perhaps the most intense level of treatment involves one-on-one work directly with a psychiatrist. These professionals have a more expansive tool kit at their fingertips than a psychologist or counselor does. The most notable example is that psychiatrists can prescribe medications. In fact, patients are often referred to psychiatrists because medication seems to be an option worth pursuing. In many cases, this type of therapy can involve significant out-of-pocket costs, so not everyone who gets a referral pursues this treatment path. When it came to medication, I was wary of side effects. But I was also looking for relief. I needed balance, both internally and in my relationships, and I believed that I owed it to myself to pursue every available option of achieving it. I was put on a variety of antianxiety medications and antidepressants as we went through the trial and error process of finding what blend of medications would work best for me. That period of experimentation wasn't the result of any doctor's incompetence; it's often how psychiatry works. You start with one prescription, and if that doesn't yield favorable results, you try a different dose or another medication. Everyone's unique, so some trial and error is an uncomfortable but necessary part of the process.

For me personally, the most effective therapeutic tool has proven to be meditation. Practicing nonreligious meditative techniques and something called "mindfulness" has helped me tremendously. Being aware of my thoughts and feelings gives me more power to keep them from controlling me. In this way, I can keep my behavior from tipping too far in any one direction. Limiting my own negative emotions is a lot easier, because I've had so much practice at this point with becoming aware of a thought or an emotion and setting it aside. Awareness of how interactions are affecting me also helps me make better decisions. Being mindful of my emotions spiking or taking a bad turn warns me that being around a certain person or doing a specific activity is negatively influencing my attitude. And that lets me ease away from situations that would send my entire day down a dark path. Part of meditation's appeal to me is that the effort and the rewards are both in my own hands. I like to have that feeling of being in control of my situation; I'm not looking to someone else to fix things for me. There are no prescriptions to fill, no side effects, and no extra personnel or equipment necessary. I can meditate when and where I need to, and that fits into my life. In other words, it works for me.

There are quite a number of tools a counselor or therapist may be able to recommend for you, including sound therapy, light therapy, and meditation, to name just a few. The modern set of therapeutic tools is quite advanced, and I can't stress highly enough the potential benefits of exploring your options. I've seen a lot of people not address their scars. They'll think, "This is just the way I am now," and settle into a life that is far less than it could be. I am a living example of how you can work through your mental or emotional scars. Whatever the issue, I want you to know that there are tools and solutions out there waiting for you to try them out. The scars you develop as you go through treatment and recovery are highly individualized, and so will be the ways you move past them. Explore whatever options seem to be a good match for what you need.

Whether you are meditating, talking in therapy sessions, or just reliably taking your meds, your progress rests in your own hands. In my experience, it wasn't uncommon to hear from a psychologist: "There is nothing more I can do for you." They had diagnosed what was happening, offered me some tools to manage the problem, and then it was up to me. And that's really what my experience with therapy has taught me. Going through all of those steps, all the various methods, and seeking guidance and the assistance of the medical community taught me that the answer ultimately doesn't come from other people. What makes those people and methods valuable is that they're there with the tools and knowledge to support us as we work through our issues. For me, making a one-, three-, and six-month goal sheet was, and continues to be, useful. Despite setting those timelines, I also needed to remember that the length of the journey wasn't the most important thing. What was and continues to be important for me, as I imagine it might be for you, too, is to make those scars manageable.

* * *

It's just as important to have a vision for the time ahead of us as it was to have a Life Plan during treatment. Think of it like this: in the very beginning, you *chose to live*. Each of us did. We were alive before, but it was a default setting. The difference between being alive and choosing to live can be as profound as the difference between someone who was simply born into a nation versus a new immigrant who worked through all the legal and other channels to gain citizenship. Either may have an appreciation for the place they live. However, the one who *chose* the history, language, and customs of a nation in order to be a part of its culture is arguably a more active citizen because of having worked for that privilege. Choosing to live changed our perspective during treatment. Each morning we woke up was a day we decided to participate in, rather than just a day that happened to us.

That initial choice allowed us to live more consciously. We had twenty-three hours outside of treatment, and we began to think about them differently. We had to become aware of what we needed day by day to thrive rather than just survive. Taking an honest look at our habits and deciding what stayed and what needed to change yielded significant growth. Learning what moves us closer to a life we enjoy and what keeps us mired in complacency is a tremendously valuable investment in living.

If during treatment you empowered yourself to make good choices for your life, then this is a habit worth continuing. If you followed my recommendations, you discovered your truest friends and supporters and drew them closer. This support network, tested and strengthened, helped you through treatment and will continue to be an asset for the rest of your life. You protected the things you've worked so hard for and gave yourself whatever stability was possible in a time when everything could have slipped away. This should give you the knowledge that if times get tough again for whatever reason, you'll be up for the challenge. You did what was necessary to stay positive, present, and in control of your life during a period that prompts many people to check out, whatever that costs them. In various ways, you learned to take charge of what you could influence, to accept what you couldn't control, and to limit the damage to your outlook and to your most important relationships. You've gotten past the danger point, alive and intact, and what did not kill you has unquestionably made you stronger.

Now, it's more important than ever to think about how you would like your days and your life to look from this point forward.

Like everything you faced before, this, too, is no easy task. But you've gotten some practice at difficult tasks by now, so I want to tell you about two more steps beyond all the ones we've already covered that I think will allow you to create, and to follow, a vision for your future.

CLOSURE RITUALS

When cancer is in the past, it becomes necessary to find a sense of closure regarding it. What I'm recommending to you is the hard work of grieving your losses. When we lose a loved one, we go through an acknowledged grieving process. What's strange about surviving cancer is that while nobody will be sad that your cancer is dead, you may very well need to mourn.

All cultures have ritual and ceremonial practices that help the living let go or bury their dead. The body of the deceased is interred in the ground, burned, set out to sea, or disposed of in some other way. Whatever culture you call your own has practices that you can turn to in order to help yourself move forward after cancer. Maybe you'll chose to privately burn something representing your cancer in your fireplace at home, or maybe you and your friends will throw your cancer an Irish-style wake. Whatever you choose, a ritual of some sort could help you acknowledge and embrace your transition into postcancer life.

By now you know that I also happen to think putting difficulties in the past is very important. No matter what, the time you spent with cancer growing inside you and the lengths you went to in order to kill it are a very big deal. I'm twelve years cancer-free at the point of writing this. People might imagine that thinking about my time in the hospital or what I went through during that period of my life wouldn't be able to touch me anymore. It'd be a mere memory. The truth is that our experiences don't ever really go away. They have the ability to haunt us, or worse, to control our present experiences in ways that we don't want.

The truth is that even though I've worked a lot on my emotions, thinking about my lymphoma brought a lot of feelings crashing back. Telling the story of my first chemo treatment meant feeling that fear and confusion all over again. Recalling the night I almost died in the cardiac ward made me experience again how utterly alone I felt while fighting to hold onto life one inhalation at a time. I also had to relive the emotional pain of holding my wife's hand through the worst moments of her life, including watching our son who seemed to be dying in front of our eyes. I had put those things behind me, and returning to them was not pleasant. It took a toll on me. This is why I'm advising you to find a method or combination of methods that will let you put cancer as firmly in the past and out of mind as you possibly can.

I insist on this partly because if we keep coming back to these memories, we'll find ourselves forever afraid. The experiences surrounding treatment, of time spent facing our own mortality or that of a loved one, are extremely stressful. There's a heightened sense of anxiety attached even to the memories of those events. Survivors can't be healthy, functioning human beings if we're so afraid of a recurrence, or of some new cancer or other illness, that we hesitate to leave our houses. We're going to have to go on with our lives and not have constant fear. The only way that can happen is if we move beyond the difficulties we've faced and give the memories the space and time to fade.

By allowing the hardships and discomforts to drift off into distant memory, we empower ourselves to press forward and meet the life ahead of us with purpose. When my own course of treatment was complete, my personal goal was to recover the time lost during treatment. I say "lost" because I had to spend that time and energy on survival instead of on my previous goals. Afterward, I was determined to rebuild all the goals that I'd put on hold, and even expand them, taking everything to a new level.

SETTING NEW GOALS

It's important to embrace your posttreatment restart. This is the time to be the person you always wanted to be, do the things you wanted to do, and eliminate the outside interference that may have prevented your earlier life from moving in the direction you wanted.

By allowing the hardships and discomforts to drift off into distant memory, we empower ourselves to press forward and meet the life ahead of us with purpose.

There was a time in my earlier life—often I refer to it as "BC," or before cancer—when I felt that I had to control absolutely everything. I attempted to do everything myself, as much as possible, and micromanaged others. The day I started coughing up blood signaled to me that those days were over. Receiving devastating news from doctors made it clear that I had to retrain my thinking and my behavior. It wasn't easy, but like any cancer patient, I had no choice: my only option for survival was to adapt. The fight we undertake by undergoing treatment requires adopting new structures and a better approach to our days, so we can successfully navigate all the unknowns that lie in front of us.

Little did I know in the beginning how important that lesson would still be once treatment was complete. The things I've learned and shared here—the ability to prioritize, to know what is in my hands and what's not, to ask for help when I need it—these and others are highly transferrable skills that have prepared me to deal with whatever comes my way. That's true for you too. Especially if you're seeking a specific result for your life, anticipating and preparing for potential obstacles, or having a "what if" plan, can be lifesaving. Often, life coaches and psychologists encourage us to focus on the positive and reflect almost exclusively on positive thoughts. You know that I think that's a reasonable approach with a good deal of utility. However, I also think that examining a given situation, determining what can go wrong, and developing a contingency plan for the outcomes with high likelihood is also a smart approach. Knowing how you would proceed should obstacles arise can lower anxiety that comes from thinking about those potential obstacles becoming realities. Instead, you can take comfort knowing that you have alternative plans for when things don't go as you imagined.

* * *

In winning your battle with cancer, you've likely realized that there's more in you than you might have previously thought. Instead of resting on those laurels, I say build on them. Use what you've just been through and the accomplishment of beating cancer as a leaping-off point. Take the skills you've learned and the inner strength you've found and move on to new accomplishments. Set yourself a new challenge, and use everything that got you through treatment to go after that goal.

When I recovered from treatment, I found myself wondering, "What now?" I didn't want to just settle back into being comfortable. Please believe that I understand the impulse. Treatment is exhausting, and we just want things to be easy for a while. Some folks want to put their feet up and relax. They'll say, "I survived cancer. That's all the difficulty I need for a while." And that's okay, for a little while.

Certainly, we all need to take the necessary time to recover enough to get back on our feet. What I want to urge against is getting too comfortable taking it easy. You just beat cancer. You're on a roll! Now you need to maintain the effort, and keep the successes coming.

That's exactly what I did: I found a way to build on my successes and grow my legacy. Lorenzo and I have recently completed renovating a building that was once a church, turning it into a fitness club. The Church, as we call it, has been a huge project, and I was spending most of my free time there. Together, Lorenzo and I found our inner strength and tested our patience and skills in order to rebuild his future. I encourage you to take advantage of whatever opportunities will help bring satisfaction to your life and mold your future in ways you never even thought possible.

This is my personal challenge to you: don't let any future simply roll out in front of you or let it be a future that someone else chose for you. Take life in hand, and shape it into what you want it to be. Take some smart risks. By now, you've already beaten worse odds than those ahead of you. I know you have what it takes to address anything that stands in your way. Any cancer survivor who doesn't yet realize that about himself or herself needs to face how strong they've really become.

What could you possibly reach for now that will be harder to attain than what you've just pulled off? I don't know what's next for you, but I can bet that you already have some ideas. There's nothing like being stuck in bed or at home for a long time to daydream about what you'd rather be doing. Now is the time to take a good look at your daydreams and pick one or two that you can see coming true if you put in the effort. It's time for your actual life to reflect your dreams.

Any time I ask a veteran survivor what their biggest fears are, a majority will answer that there isn't much to be afraid of anymore.

They'll explain that the fear that once kept them from facing uncomfortable situations is far easier to overcome. Leaps of faith they always used to shy away from are now much easier to make. When someone is young and chasing after their dreams, most people roll their eyes and wait for them to fail. They figure that since most lives are mediocre, why should this kid's be any different? But it doesn't matter what those people think because you've already stopped giving them power to affect you. My guess is that the rest of the world will be a little in awe as you dust yourself off and move forward toward your goals. They'll see that what I'm telling you is true: whatever goal you set yourself now will be a small thing compared to what you just accomplished.

Now it's time for you to choose what comes next in your story and to go make it amazing.

Be prepared for people to view you a little differently. Now you're a bit like an action hero in a movie walking away from a flaming car crash. The wreckage is burning behind you, and you're not looking back because you have places to be. You have dreams and ambitions to make real. You're far from finished with life.

Now it's time for you to choose what comes next in your story and to go make it amazing.